Bella Mack ... *Jog On* is her f ...

Praise for *Jog On*

...mely and empathetic . . . an ins... ...on what it's like
...perience, and confront one's ...tal health . . . warm,
...ible and perfect.'                                                    *Grazia*

...k of real hope and one that will truly inspire you.'
                                                                                      *Stylist*

...'s brilliant love letter to running turns into an extraordinarily
...e and frank account of her battle with anxiety. This is a
...passionate and important book which presents running as a
...ble but effective antidote to an anxious world.'          Joe Lycett

...insightful take on what it's like to experience, and confront
...'s mental health while joyfully celebrating the fact that just
...ing an everyday runner can be enough to change your life.
...arm, accessible and perfect for resetting a glum January
...ndset.' Alexandra Heminsley, author of *Running Like a Girl*

...heartfelt and joyous ode to the strange, wonderful pull of a
...r of ugly trainers, tight fitting Polyyester, the rainy, windy
...en road and the peace and clarity it brings. Anyone that runs
...ll love this book.'                                            Dermot O'Leary

...don't know that I will ever become a runner but this book is
...inspiring start to the year.'                          Nigella Lawson

...*g On* will act as a comfort – and a spur –. to so many. It is
kind, it is honest and it will make you finally pull on those
trainers and get moving. It will also – and this is so important
– help you to understand what those experiencing anxiety
endure.'                                                            Lynn Enright

Also by Bella Mackie

*Jog On Journal: A Practical Guide to
Getting Up and Running*

BELLA MACKIE

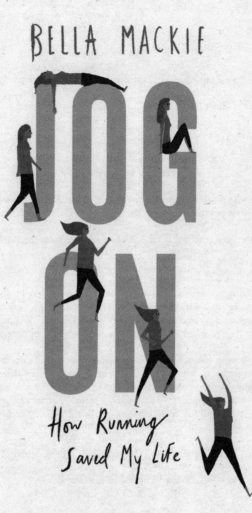

JOG ON

How Running Saved My Life

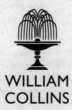

WILLIAM
COLLINS

William Collins
An imprint of HarperCollins*Publishers*
1 London Bridge Street
London SE1 9GF

WilliamCollinsBooks.com

First published in Great Britain in 2018 by William Collins

This William Collins paperback edition published in 2019

1

ISBN 978-0-00-824172-8

Set in Garamond Pro by
Palimpsest Book Production Ltd, Falkirk, Stirlingshire

Printed and bound in Great Britain by
CPI Group (UK) Ltd, Croydon CR0 4YY

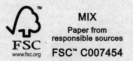

MIX
Paper from
responsible sources
FSC™ C007454

FSC
www.fsc.org

This book is produced from independently certified FSC™ paper
to ensure responsible forest management.

For more information visit: www.harpercollins.co.uk/green

For George,
who was as brave as anyone I ever met,
and to whom I owe most things.

# CONTENTS

1K — EVERYTHING IS AWFUL

I ran for three minutes today. In the dark, slowly, and not all in one go. That's three minutes more than I've ever run in my life. I'm out of breath and I've got a stitch and I already feel better than I have in years. That's enough for a first attempt. Now I can go back home and have a cry. Or some wine.

Even as I lay on the floor of my sitting room, watching my husband's feet walking quickly towards the door, I was already thinking about what was to come. When a marriage breaks down, there will be unbearable sadness, awkward questions, sometimes embarrassment. I could imagine all of them. Staring down at the rug, my mind had jumped ahead, blurrily plotting out the impending future. I even started to vaguely compile the inevitable playlist of terrible songs that I knew would be belting out mournfully at 4 a.m. for weeks to come.

I have learnt now that the actual moment of heartbreak can be astonishingly brief. It's not always the drawn-out disintegration you imagine it might be as an adult, bits of love and comfort slowly breaking off over years, until there's nothing left to say at all. Sometimes it happens in a flash, takes you by surprise, gives you no time to prepare. Someone stands across from you, looks directly into your eyes and tells you that they are leaving you, that they no longer love you, that they have found someone else, that you are not enough, and you think: 'Oh, so this is the moment that I am going to die. I can't possibly get through this.' Somewhere, something in your body has savagely ruptured, and all you can think to do is to lie down on the floor and wait to be invited to walk down the inevitable tunnel of light.

I don't know which way is worse. Both are hideous, most break-ups are. I once heard a story about a couple in a restaurant who ate in total silence for over an hour. When coffee came, the husband whispered something to the wife, who hissed back: 'It's not the coffee, it's the last twenty-five years.' A slow crumbling like that would be pretty appalling. But when you're given the surprise approach, the moment of impact feels brutally physical. Despite this shock, it's also, weirdly, the easy bit. Because sooner or later, you realise that you're not going to die. And you can't even stare blankly at the carpet for too long because you have to pick up your kids from school, or walk the dog, or go to work. Maybe you just need to pee. Your pain doesn't even stand up to the most mundane demands of an idle Monday. And after this unwelcome realisation, you see the future quite clearly: you'll stumble through this moment. But it takes such a long time. Heartbreak is brief. The way out of it is interminable, and sometimes you resent even having to try.

Even as I lay there, I knew that I would shortly have to get up off the floor. I even knew that, with the right coping skills, it might be OK in the end. But I also knew something else. I knew that unlike most adults, I didn't have any coping skills.

We learn to feel long before we learn how to make sense

of those feelings. Babies laugh and cry, and get angry, yet can't tell us why. But as we grow up, we develop the methods we need to help us deal with stressful or traumatic events. Our teenage years are often spent feeling frustrated and confused, but we eventually gain insight into ourselves, and we learn how to better deal with mature emotions. We take these tools with us into adulthood, where we refine them and grow to develop a clearer understanding of how to face our own personal challenges. At least, most of us do. But right up until the moment I found myself lying on the floor, I had spent a lifetime running away from my problems. Anxious even as a very small child, I had let my worries fester, take control, and dominate my life. Mental-health problems had stunted my own growth, leaving me too scared to take on challenges, trying to rigidly control the environment around me to prevent any possible hurt. Quitting things when they got hard. Turning down opportunities that would push me, or give me independence. Being small.

I got used to hiding my head in the sand from a young age, and using magical thinking to ward off bad things. Instead of recognising I was ill, I'd come up with ways to cope with my worries and irrational thoughts, none of them successful. I'd spit if I had a scary idea, or blink hard to expel it. I'd avoid certain numbers, letters, colours, songs and places. All as a way to 'compromise' with my brain, in the hopes that the bad thoughts would go away if I just stuck rigidly to my little mechanisms. Nothing worked, and my anxiety mushroomed. My coping skills were all false friends and, as a consequence, I was agoraphobic, prone to panic attacks, intrusive thoughts, hysteria and depression. By the time my husband walked out on me, I'd had years of this. I (honestly) couldn't make it to the supermarket on my own, much less navigate my way through a break-up of this magnitude. I knew I had to get off the floor but I didn't know what to do next. Everything was draped in fear.

Anxiety is a slippery, sneaky thing. It's an illness that manifests itself in so many different ways that it's often not diagnosed until the sufferer is absolutely desperate. You might spend years having panic attacks you don't even recognise as panic attacks. You might assume that you're seriously unwell, as though you're having a stroke or a heart attack (like I did aged eighteen in a nightclub, much to the hilarity of my drunken friends), or research high blood pressure obsessively. You might be so ashamed of your intrusive thoughts that you never dare confide in anyone, let alone allow yourself to think you show signs of obsessive-compulsive disorder (OCD). Instead of dealing with the horrible images and ideas that pop into your mind, recognising that they're just thoughts and can't hurt you, you might spend years trying to neutralise and silence them. All of this can make you severely depressed, as if you don't have enough to cope with. It made me cry hysterically, it made me stay in bed for hours. It made me sleep away days. It made me watch more daytime TV than a happy person should or would. It made me lose all hope far too young.

By the time they reach this stage, a person with an anxiety disorder will likely have come up with their own mechanisms to deal with such frightening thoughts and sensations. Those coping skills will be rigid and hard to challenge, never mind break down. Almost none of these will be helpful in the long term. More often they provide some instant relief, but ultimately serve to tighten the bonds of the worry they're having.

With me, these tactics included never returning to a place where I'd had a panic attack. Sensible plan, I thought, to avoid the same horrible situation happening again. Except I ended up putting an invisible cordon around most of London, including my local high street, the park and most shops. This later widened to include planes, lifts, motorways, anywhere too far away from a hospital, and the Underground (I was a lot of fun at parties). The immediate comfort this gave me was deceptive, since I quickly found myself trapped – unable to go anywhere that my mind had designated to be 'unsafe'. Though it's clear to me now that I'd been in the grip of anxiety for many years, I was so used to my own shoddy bargaining methods that I didn't seek effective help with it until these tactics had a vice-like grip on me, and I was at a standstill.

If ever there is a trigger to make you try and change something, it's the shock of your marriage collapsing before you've even made it to a year. Given that people who get divorced in the UK have usually managed about eleven and a half years before they pull the plug, tanking your vows as spectacularly as I did felt like quite the feat. Any longer and it might just have been seen as sad, unavoidable, or chalked up to 'young people not sticking at anything anymore', but eight months? It would be unwise not to question your life just a little bit after that.

And even without the added inconvenience of a marriage breakdown, I already knew that I had reached a crunch point. I'd avoided everything I found scary for so long that my world had shrunk to the point where I felt like I was suffocating. Despite all my careful management and precautions (read controlling everything and employing wildly irrational thinking – like I say, fun at parties), the worst had happened. The framework I'd been building for myself since I was a child hadn't protected me from harm or humiliation. In fact, it had greatly contributed to it.

After my husband walked out, I'd spent several days weeping and drinking after my sister forcibly pulled me up from the foetal position I had adopted on the floor. Forgive me if I don't give any detail here – I can't remember a thing about those moments. I'm grateful to my brain for that, one of the only times it's served me well. There must have been talking, sleeping and food but all I can remember is watching an entire season of *Game of Thrones* and my sister getting angry that I'd binge-watched it without her.

I took one day off work and then went back to the office, alternately crying in the toilets (my husband worked for the same company, that was fun) and sitting mute at my desk, listening to bagpipe music on my headphones in a strange attempt to find some mettle whenever I saw him walk by. As an aside, this was strangely effective and I would recommend it to anyone needing to feel strong. Start with 'Highland Laddie'.

I felt stagnant, aware that I had to endure these painful and difficult emotions, but also worried that I might never feel truly better. Life continues around you, no matter how much your own world has been shattered. I could see normality heave into view and I didn't want it. I was back at work, and I suspected that within a few months I might be over the break-up but still locked in my small space, anxiety and depression my only real bedfellows.

It's easy to behave like nothing is wrong, even when you have a mental illness and feel like you're going to be consumed by it. Even at my most miserable, I was good at holding down my job, cracking jokes, going out just enough so I wasn't seen as a hermit. Many people become experts at this, even tricking themselves. I could probably have gone on like this forever, living half a life, pretending that I was OK with it. But something had broken, and I couldn't do it anymore. I'd done it for so long, and it had become exhausting.

I saw myself exposed as a fraud – a cowardly kid play-acting as an adult, with no business being there. J. K. Rowling says that rock bottom became the foundation upon which she built her life – that because her worst fears had been realised, she had nowhere to go but up.[1] As it's her, I can allow the cliché and even grudgingly admit that it fits. In Rowling's case, she went on to create a magical world of wizards which helped her to become one of the richest women in the world. In mine, rock bottom spurred me on to go for a jog.

One week into my newly single life, I had the idea to run. There's a moment in *The Catcher in the Rye*[2] when Holden Caulfield runs across the school playing fields and explains it away by saying: 'I don't even know what I was running for – I guess I just felt like it.' Maybe I was just fed up with feeling so damn miserable, or perhaps I already knew that I had to try and do something differently, but that day I just felt like running.

I still don't know why that was the tool I opted for in the midst of misery. I'd never done any kind of strenuous exercise before in my life. But I *had* spent a lifetime holding at bay the need to run away – from my mind, from my negative thoughts; from the worries that built up and calcified, layer upon layer, until they were too strong to chip away at. Maybe the sudden urge to run was a physical manifestation of this desire to escape my own brain. I guess I just wanted to do it for real.

Plus, I was impatient to bypass the ice-cream-binging stereo-
type of a break-up – I've always been keen for a quick fix. I
wanted the bad feelings and heartache to be gone fast. A
break-up is always a good time to try and do something new,
after all. I had the added benefit of also wanting to break free
of my lifelong fears, and I really felt like time was running
out to do that. I was about to turn thirty, and I was terrified
that I would use the break-up as another excuse to retreat, to
box myself in even more, to be scared of life itself.

I was not ready to run across a playing field by any means.
Being too scared to go to the supermarket put paid to any
grandiose ideas like that. There was no climactic movie
moment where I streaked across a prairie or raced through a
downpour. In reality, I didn't know what I was doing and I
fleetingly wondered if I was in fact becoming delusional. It
seemed like such a strange thing for me to want to do, and
yet even as I argued with myself, I was gathering my keys and
lacing up my trainers.

I put on some old leggings and a T-shirt and walked to a
dark alleyway thirty seconds from my flat. It fitted two important criteria: just near enough to the safety of home, and just
quiet enough that nobody would laugh at me. I felt absurd
and slightly ashamed – as if I was doing something perverse
that shouldn't be seen. Luckily, the only sign of life was a cat
who stared at me disdainfully as I mustered up the energy to
move. I was grateful when the cat immediately vanished; and
any hint of an approaching human would have made me stop
instantly. This kind of private punishment was too raw to be
seen by strangers.

With my headphones in, I searched for suitable music and
settled upon a song called 'She Fucking Hates Me' by a band

called Puddle of Mudd. Not to my usual taste, but the lyrics were suitably angry and I didn't want anything that might make me cry (everything was making me cry). The song is three minutes and thirty-one seconds long and the line 'she fucking hates me' comes up as many times as you might imagine. I think I managed thirty seconds of jogging before I had to stop, calves screaming and lungs burning. But the song was kicking off my adrenaline and so I rested for a minute, and then started off again. I somehow managed to keep time with the shouting singer, mouthing the words as I screwed up my face and lumbered down the path. I managed an incredible three minutes in stages (nearly all the song!) before I gave up and went home. Did I feel better? No. Did I enjoy it? Also no, but I hadn't cried for at least fifteen minutes and that was good enough for me.

To my own surprise, I didn't leave it there. I wanted to, it had felt pretty grim, but something in me overrode all my internal excuses. I went back to that same alley the next day. And the day after that. Those first few attempts were all pathetic really. A few seconds, shuffle, stop. Wait. Go again. Freeze if a person emerged from the shadows. Feel ridiculous. Carry on anyway. Always in the dark, always in secret, as if I was somehow transgressing.

I didn't know what I was doing, or what I wanted to get out of these alley runs. As a result, I got overly ambitious in the following weeks, and I encountered frequent and minor disasters. I got shin splints, which hurt like hell. I ran too fast and had to stop after wheezing uncontrollably. I tried to go up a hill and had to admit defeat and get on a bus when it became clear that the hill had bested me; I had a panic attack in a dark part of the local park when I mistimed sunset and realised that I was all alone. I fell over and cried like a child. Running felt like a language that I couldn't speak – and not only because I was hugely unfit – it seemed to be something that only happy healthy bouncy people did, not neurotic smokers who were scared of everything.

Throughout my life, if I couldn't do something well on the first attempt, I was prone to quit almost immediately. It was embarrassingly clear to me that I was not running well, or getting better at it. And yet, much to my own quiet disbelief, I carried on. I carried on trudging up and down the dark alleyway for two weeks. And when I finally felt bored rather than just merely terrified or out of breath, I went a little bit further. For the first couple of months, I stuck to the roads closest to my flat – my brain always looking for the escape route – looping around quiet streets, and cringing when cars passed by. I was slow, sad and angry. But two things were becoming clear to me. The first was that when I ran I didn't feel quite so sad. My mind would quieten down – some part of my brain seemed to switch off, or at least cede control for a few minutes. I wouldn't think about my marriage, or my part in its failure. I wouldn't wonder if my husband was happy, or out on a great date, or just not thinking about me at all. The relief this gave me was immense.

The second thing, which was even more valuable, was that I noticed that I wasn't feeling so anxious. Soon enough, I was reaching parts of the city that I hadn't been able to visit in years, especially alone. I mean, I'm not talking the centre of Soho and its bustling crowds, but within a month I was able to run through the markets of Camden without feeling like I would faint or break down. I could not have done this if I'd been walking – I'd tried so many times but my anxiety would break through, palms sweating and looming panic taking over. But somehow, running was different. When your brain has denied you the chance to take the mundane excursions that most people do every day, being able to pass through stalls selling 'nobody knows I'm a lesbian' T-shirts suddenly feels like a red-letter day. By concentrating on the rhythm of my feet striking the pavement, I wasn't obsessing over my breathing, or the crowds, or how far I was from home. I could be in an area my brain had previously designated as 'unsafe', and not feel like I was going to faint. It was miraculous to me.

Joyce Carol Oates once described how running enables her writing, positing that it helps as 'the mind flies with the body'.[3] I take that to mean that your body takes your brain along for the ride. Your mind is no longer in the driving seat. You're concentrating on the burn in your legs, the swing of your arms. You notice your heartbeat, the sweat dripping into your ears, the way your torso twists as you stride. Once you're in a rhythm, you start to notice obstacles in your way, or people to avoid. You see details on buildings you'd never noticed before. You anticipate the weather ahead of you. Your brain has a role in all of this, but not the role it is used to. My mind, accustomed to frightening me with endless 'what if' thoughts, or happy to torment me with repeated flashbacks to my worst experiences, simply could not compete with the need to concentrate while moving fast. I'd tricked it, or exhausted it, or just given it something new to deal with.

Much research has been done on why running clears your head so effectively. Scientists seem intent on finding out why it works. I'm glad they are – I'd like to know exactly why running changed my life, but honestly I'm mainly just happy that it *has*. Studies have found that there is an increased activity in the brain's frontal lobe after activity – the area linked to focus and concentration – in subjects with mild cognitive impairment and in elderly participants.[45] Research on animals has shown that exercise produces new neurons – cells found in the hippocampus, associated with memory and learning.[6] It's all fascinating stuff. But to my mind, none of this can adequately convey the rush that exercise promises to give you – that's the main interest to most of us – the so-called runner's high. (People with more experience with drugs than I have had will have to judge whether it is comparable to a more, er, recreational experience.) That an hour or so of energetic movement a day might fix our stressed and gloomy heads is understandably alluring, especially to those of us who've struggled with depression or anxiety for a sustained (read intolerable) period of time.

This is what I was beginning to dip my toes into. Weeks after my marriage collapsed, I was still sick with it all. At work, I would regularly go into the toilets and cry quietly. At home, I would put on my pyjamas the moment I got in and mindlessly watch whatever the TV had to offer. When I went out, I drank too much and would cry again (less quietly this time, to the delight of my friends). But when I ran, I left it all behind. Nobody could give me the dreaded sympathy head-tilt or an excruciating hug. Nobody even looked at me. I melted into the city, another tiresome runner in hi-vis. At home, I felt desperately lonely. I'd taken to sleeping like a starfish to head off the inevitable moment in the morning where I'd roll over and be met with a cold empty space, a reminder of all I'd lost. But when I headed out in the morning to run, I didn't feel alone. I soon found that I was setting myself little challenges – go two minutes further today, run down that busy road that you've avoided for years tomorrow. The more I did it, the more I found that I was rediscovering the city that I lived in and yet barely understood – for so long a place fraught with imagined danger for me. I ran down Holloway Road looking at the tops of the faded old buildings that housed convenience stores and supermarkets. I discovered railway lines that ran like arteries through built-up estates, hidden from plain sight. I ran along the canal and found an expanse of brambles, wild flowers and baby ducklings swimming along next to me. The panic attacks were fading away. Not once did I feel the need to find the exit; my feet were in control and I was running purposefully, not running away. I was taking things in for the first time without my mind screaming warnings at me.

It would be taking things too far to say that I felt childlike when I ran, but it definitely gave me a sense of lightness and abandon that I only really see in young people (and drunk people, but they then have a sense of regret which I hope children don't experience). This shouldn't be a surprise; from an early age we are encouraged to skip, hop, dance, run and play team sports. As Louisa May Alcott wrote: 'Active exercise was my delight from the time when a child of six I drove my hoop around the Common without stopping, to the days when I did my twenty miles in five hours and went to a party in the evening. I always thought I must have been a deer or a horse in some former state, because it was such a joy to run.'[7] We instinctively know that the young need to use their bodies, and not only for their physical health. Studies on this in the UK are somewhat limited, and usually cross-sectional, but a NICE study on children and exercise remarked on the results of one survey which reported a higher risk of depressive symptoms among 933 eight- to twelve-year-olds classified as inactive, and among children not meeting the standards for health-related fitness compared with those who were considered active.[8] Analysis of clinical trials looking at exercise and its effect on depressive symptoms in teens aged thirteen to seventeen seemed to show that physical exercise is an effective treatment strategy.[9]

I never gave myself the chance to learn this when I was younger. It would be simplistic to say that this was all because of anxiety, although it was certainly a contributing factor. I was chubby, rather unpopular and viewed sport as a hideous popularity contest. I hope that things have changed since I was at primary school, but sports were also determined by gender. You almost never saw girls on the football pitch, and it was perfectly acceptable for us to gather in sedentary groups around the playground as the boys burnt off their energy kicking a ball about. The divide is still marked – a 2013 study found that half of British seven-year-olds don't get enough exercise, and the gap between boys and girls was one of the most worrying revelations.[10] Professor Carol Dezateux, one of the lead authors on the study, said of the findings: 'There is a big yawning gap between girls and boys. We need to really think about how we are reaching out to girls . . . The school playground is an important starting point. Often you will find it dominated by boys playing football.'

The rate of exercise drops by as much as 40 per cent as children move through primary school.[11] And this decline didn't stop for me at secondary school, where we were marched down to a sodden field to play hockey (I told you it was gendered, netball was the only other option). I would inevitably be picked last and then proceed to stand as far away from the action as possible. As we got a bit older, our options for exercise were an unaccompanied walk round the local park, or aerobics. Given that the park contained a) boys and b) cigarettes, guess where I went?

Women in Sport recently conducted research into the variation between girls' and boys' levels of exercise, and they found that just 12 per cent of girls aged fourteen got enough physical activity every week.[12] [13] Despite this dismal number, 76 per cent of fifteen-year-old girls said that they would like to do more physical activity but were discouraged by the sports on offer to them. The other (and to my mind, sadder) reason that they gave for not participating was that they thought that sport was 'unfeminine'. I remember that feeling clearly – a sense that exercise was just not dignified or elegant. It involved sweat and grunting and angry screwed-up faces, and could well end up in embarrassment, a thing all teenagers wisely (or perhaps just instinctively?) avoid like the plague.

As children leave full-time education, exercise rates can decline further. Sure, some will make time for a run or a gym session, but it gets harder. If you end up going to university, it's unlikely you'll be making time for sport when there's so much work to do and terrible fancy dress parties to attend. There's a reason why people gloomily talk about the 'Freshers' Fifteen' – the old but accurate cliché that you put on weight in the first year of studying. This mirrored my experience, where activity meant getting out of bed past midday and possibly walking to the local shop for fags and crisps. A fairly normal experience for a student then, except that, unfortunately, this is also the age when some anxiety disorders are known to manifest themselves most severely – for example, OCD usually develops before the age of twenty.[14] While aspects of anxiety will be present in kids from a much younger age (phobias show up in children as young as seven), early adulthood is the perfect time for more serious aspects of anxiety and depression to hit, and hit hard. And that shouldn't be surprising to anyone – after all, this is the time when the carefully regimented structures of education and family fall away and you are mostly in charge for the first time. Some thrive with the new responsibilities that they've been given, but many will not. I did not.

Having managed to leave school with most of my childish worries lying fairly dormant, I was knocked off my feet one day at university, when, completely out of the blue, I had a terrible panic attack in a courtyard. I was so unprepared for these feelings to rear up on me again that I deployed my trusty ostrich manoeuvre and tried to ignore it. Instead of questioning why it had happened, I simply avoided all thought of it. But the feelings of rising panic increased in a frighteningly short period of time, and within a fortnight I had developed a new symptom which horrified me more than any I had previously experienced: disassociation. The clever (not a compliment) thing about anxiety is that the moment you've got a handle on one thing (night sweats, panic attacks, dizziness, nausea, headaches – come sit by me), it'll throw you another one, and you better believe it'll be worse.

Disassociation (or derealisation) is a condition which makes the world suddenly seem unreal. Actually, I don't think I've made this sound as heart-stoppingly awful as it is. It's not just the world that feels unreal – it's that the people you love the most seem fake, your home feels like a film set, your dog looks flat, your own face doesn't look like your face. Everything feels staged and wrong and just . . . off. I later learnt that psychiatrists believe that it's a sensation your brain employs when it's exhausted from worrying – shutting your mind down (somewhat). So it's actually an attempt at protection, but to me it feels a bit like a mate who sleeps with your partner and earnestly explains that they only did it to help you. I'm not saying thank you either way.

What would have happened if I'd just put on some trainers and tried to outrun these awful feelings? It's something I've asked myself repeatedly in the years since. Nothing is as simple as that, and it would be insulting and irresponsible to even hint that it could be. Running is not a cure-all for severe mental illness, or anything else for that matter. It's right to acknowledge that early on. But I often think of the girl I was in my twenties and wish I could go back and try other things, as many of my friends did when things got difficult. Your twenties are a time for experimenting, having fun and enjoying everything that life may offer you, or so we're told. Instead, for many people, I think they are a time of massive insecurity, debt, and a sense of displacement – a decade of worry and fear. So I did what I could. I dropped out of Uni, went to a psychiatrist and took the antidepressants that I was swiftly prescribed. What else could I do? At this point, suicidal thoughts were creeping in, and even through my wildly unreal prism, I could tell that those thoughts would only lead somewhere I didn't want to think about in further detail.

Despite all of this, I was extremely fortunate – it's so important that I recognise that. I had a family who, while not fully understanding at all why their daughter was crying hysterically all the time and refusing to go out, had the resources to pay for me to see a professional. Seventy-eight per cent of students reported a mental-health issue in 2015, and 33 per cent of those had suicidal thoughts.[15] My NHS GP was kind, but could only offer to put me on the waiting list for therapy, which stood at six months back then. More than one in ten people currently wait over a year for any kind of talking therapy, with the same number having to scrape together the private funds to pay for help themselves. Some universities are now offering exercise classes (in tandem with the usual talking therapies) to students with depression and anxiety, an encouraging sign that experts in mental health are still linking up the physical and the mental in ways we've not yet fully explored.

It's not just depression and anxiety that an activity like running has been proven to help with. Even as you read this, you might well be experiencing something equally as isolating: you might be feeling lonely. Loneliness is something that we increasingly recognise has a huge impact on our mental and physical health, yet so many people still feel unable to admit to it. The stigma that surrounds it can make us feel pathetic, unlikeable, inadequate, and it can be really hard to see a way out of it. People often say it's hard to walk alone in life. Sometimes it's bloody hard to run alone too. This may be why Parkrun has become such a hit across the UK. Every week, at 414 parks scattered around the country (and in fourteen countries worldwide), people congregate early in the morning to jog together.[16] Though I often need to run alone, some of the best routes I have taken have been with my sister, with an ex-boyfriend and with new friends, where we've shuffled along, gradually getting to know one another better while pushing each other forwards. When you're unable to put on a front because you're wheezing and sweating profusely, it's genuinely astonishing how close you can feel to the person next to you doing the same.

As I was writing this book, a survey of more than 8,000 people was carried out by Glasgow Caledonian University to look at whether running can make you happier. The questionnaire used the Oxford Happiness Questionnaire, and asked people to answer questions using a rating between 1 (unhappy) and 6 (extremely happy). Parkrun participants emerged with an average of 4.4, compared to the general population, who scored an average 4.[17] The sense of community that running with others provides ranked highly with the responders, who said that the support and sociable elements of running with others was invaluable.

Sara, who suffered with postnatal depression after the birth of her first child, told me that running with a friend provided some light in the dark. Someone who would pick her up and force her out, someone who pushed her on and kept her going when she might not have bothered herself.

'I'm quite a solo runner, and a bit of a hermit, so I actually like running by myself and get a lot of benefit from that, but at the same time I know the fact that I had one friend who kept pushing me (in a nice way) to run was probably a key part of my recovery that one time,' she told me. 'I might've done it myself eventually, but she certainly speeded things along. And, of course, having meaningful connections with other people is a big part of sustaining good mental health. I've always felt that it's the physical act which is key for me, because I get kind of addicted to the physical sensations, but actually I realise now that without that key friend I might not have managed to get that far!'

So many people I spoke to during the course of writing this book spoke of the important social aspect that running provides. Running with a partner, or a friend, or just meeting people out and about can be a balm to the isolation that mental-health problems create. Even if you run alone, you're connecting with the world around you, and it's still surprising just how effective that can be when you've not spoken to another person in days.

Alongside the effect exercise can have on depression and anxiety, there have been some amazing clinical trials that have looked into whether aerobic exercise can help people who suffer from schizophrenia. A 2016 study at the University of Manchester reported that working out reduced the symptoms in patients with psychosis by 27 per cent.[18] Initial trials in the USA on veterans with post-traumatic stress disorder (PTSD) have also found that exercise brings about a reduction in fear, along with a lessening of the physical symptoms. Of course, all these results do not negate the need for therapy, medication and other support structures, but they bring hope that there is perhaps also more that we can do to help ourselves.

The pills that I took definitely helped, and I was able to look at myself in a mirror again without wondering who the fuck was looking back at me. I got a job, was able to go out again (while always looking for the fire escapes), and managed a few relationships. I was patched up, in the most basic sense. Nothing was fixed, but I wasn't staring at walls and hyper-ventilating either, so I took the pill. I say all this, not to give you a small insight into my not particularly special mind, but to show how easy it is to accept the most pallid imitations of existence when you've got a mental illness. To paint on a small canvas, and to pretend that you're happy with the narrow perimeters you're able to move within. Not at all a life wasted by any means, but a life limited in a variety of ways. It can feel just about fine, but it can also feel stunted, a compromise that takes a lot from you. So to find something that breaks you free of this can feel utterly miraculous. For some that may mean medication, for others meditation. My mother does yoga whenever she feels low. A colleague of mine lifts weights to keep depression at bay, and one friend boxes because he feels far too angry and it helps keep those thoughts under control. One girl I know with severe bipolar credits her treks across the local park with saving her in small ways every day. I even know somebody who cross-stitches when she feels that familiar anxiety rushing in. Somehow, after a decade of settling for merely 'managing', I'd found the thing that broke me out of it: I'd found running.

One day, after a few months of gingerly testing myself trudging around the local streets that I'd come to know with my feet, I decided to go further. I ran to my firmly set boundaries, and then I ran past them. I ran into the heart of the city, towards one of the bridges that traverse the Thames and beckon you over with the promise of light and air, and I headed across without a backwards glance. I crossed another bridge, intoxicated by the sunshine on my skin, and I ran into Parliament Square, thronging with the usual tourists and vendors and honking cars. I passed through Soho, marvelling at the noise and the rickshaws and the sex shops. I kept going, like a neurotic Forrest Gump, until I physically couldn't go any further. And when I stopped, I wandered around. The pit in my stomach wasn't raw, I wasn't checking my breathing – I didn't notice my body at all. I was able to take in my surroundings and enjoy them. I felt triumphant. I felt . . . happy.

When you do something that allows you a respite from misery, it can be hard not to get addicted to it. We all know that just as a person who uses drugs and alcohol can quickly become dependent on them, and in a different way, the same can be said of exercise. The rush I experienced that made me feel so happy that day in central London can be hard to say goodbye to, even briefly. Once you've found something that makes you feel halfway to normal, why would you *not* step it up? After all, exercise is healthy – we're constantly being told to do more of it by our doctors, the media and now increasingly by Instagram stars and vloggers who preach about clean eating and physical exertion. But for someone who is looking for a crutch, or a way to feel less lost, exercise can move quite quickly from enabling you to dominating you. Although there are comparatively few studies on exercise addiction, one from 2012 found that 3 per cent of gym-goers fit the description of an addict, and another study suggested that number might be more like 25 per cent for amateur runners.[19] It can be extremely hard to notice when something that you feel is doing you good begins to take over your life.

Every person will have their own measure for how much is too much, but my criteria would include the following: Would you say no to a night out because you don't want a hangover before a big workout? What about never having lunch with colleagues because you use that time to run? Or might you get panicky when there's a weekend wedding coming up because you worry that you'll miss a gym session? I would have to reluctantly say yes to two of these questions (I will absolutely run through a hangover, come on), because at times, running has unquestionably become an obsession for me. The utter joy I found in the absence of panic attacks, irrational thoughts and all the other symptoms that anxiety brings with it (there are over a hundred, just try to beat me) was intoxicating. Feel that heady haze often enough and it becomes easy to turn down other things. Online, you'll quickly find countless stories of people who have made very real sacrifices in their lives to maintain their exercise routine – people doing workouts three times a day, those who would panic if they missed a cycle or a swim but became exhausted from the commitment. And this goes against what the person hoped it would do in the beginning. Running was something that allowed me to have a life – a real life, with friends and new experiences and even risk. It was a wonderful means to an end, but it was never meant to be my whole life.

After a life lived in varying degrees of fear, once you feel as though you've managed to find an even keel, you guard it fiercely. Any normal sign of panic or a fleeting feeling of doom can knock you off your perch – making you worried that you're going to be sent straight back to square one, do not pass go. In those moments, I would step up my routine – putting on my trainers twice a day, pushing myself harder. At times like this I hated running. I felt like a hamster willingly signing up to a new wheel, but now unable to get off. I might have continued in this vein, were it not for something catastrophic that happened less than a year after my husband had pushed off. The woman that I loved as a second mother, the woman who gave me my first job, and taught me how to be an adult, and hugged me and laughed at me and screeched at my gossip: she died. She died far too young, and she took with her a joy that I haven't seen in anyone since. In the days and weeks afterwards, as those left behind began to understand just what had been taken from us, we were enveloped in sorrow. I ran, hoping to ameliorate the grief, hoping that my fail-safe would do what it had been doing for the past nine

months. And it helped, it truly did. You find it hard to cry
when you run – for one thing, I think you'd end up feeling
like you were in a music video from the nineties, weeping as
you dashed through a downpour wearing something bedazzling
– and running forces you to understand, in the most literal
sense, that the world keeps moving even when you think it
shouldn't, even when you're furious that it does. I'm not the
first to use running to try and get over a great loss – the
world's oldest marathon runner, Fauja Singh (a sprightly 107),
started running in his late eighties to get over the loss of his
wife and children.

But while running provided a balm, an event of such
horrible magnitude also showed me that it had its limitations.
And that was something I needed to learn. I'm loath to say
that the loss of a much loved friend can bring about anything
positive. It just can't. But I did come to understand that you
should not fear real sadness, nor try to shy away from it. And
that doesn't mean that you'll fall down the rabbit hole of
mental illness again, nor that you'll never recover. You can't
fully insulate yourself against true sorrow, but you can learn
to recognise the difference between a natural and worthy
emotion like grief, and an irrational and unhealthy one, like
panic. I scaled back my escalating running schedule and
allowed myself to feel sad sometimes. By doing that, I remembered why I had come to love doing it so much.

Running is not magic beans and I now know that I can't
expect it to inure me to the genuine sadness of life. But
throughout tough periods in my life, and without realising it,
I had finally acquired a coping skill, one that has helped me
every day since I found myself on that floor, wondering how
I'd ever get up. It's something that has taken me out of my

self-made cage, propelled me towards new jobs, new experiences, real love and a sense of optimism and confidence that I can be more than just a woman with crippling anxiety. It has given me a new identity, one which no longer sees danger and fear first. It's not an exaggeration to say that I ran myself out of misery. It has transformed my life.

# 2K - IN SICKNESS AND IN HEALTH

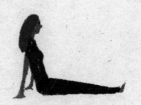

I'm running a loop of three local roads. I can't go any further in case I have a panic attack. I have to stick near safety. I'm so slow that I'm overtaken by a dog walker as I go, and I stop every minute or so, as my lungs burn and my shins ache. Voices in my head whisper conflicting things: 'Go on, this run is going better than yesterday.' 'Why are you bothering to do this? You're really bad at it.' And the meanest of all: 'This won't make your husband love you, you know.' That one sticks and mutates: 'You've failed. Anxiety is your companion, stop trying to fight it off. Aren't you embarrassed about how your life has ended up?' I'm trying to shake these relentless thoughts off, but it's hard. My eyes feel funny and my arms feel shaky. I ask myself my daily question – is this anxiety or something worse? I don't know. I just know my body is hurting and I feel useless. My legs are heavy, and I feel jittery. I manage twelve minutes and go home, wondering if I can do it again when it feels so hard.

This book is not about a great love affair gone awry. Writing it many years after the breakdown of my marriage almost feels fraudulent, since it was so brief, and in hindsight, such a huge mistake. Viewing it from a decent distance, I see it as a blip, and not even a blip I think about much. But it wasn't something to totally regret, because it forced me to acknowledge that something much bigger and much worse needed to be tackled. It was merely a catalyst to get me to deal with anxiety, so I'm grateful for it in a way. In a very weird, weird way. It's also a different kind of love story – cue swelling music – one about loving myself.

Since much of this book will be about anxiety, it might be helpful to look at just what that word means. What it really *means*. Because the worries you have on an idle Sunday evening do not constitute an anxiety disorder. And that's no bad thing! Feeling anxious from time to time is totally normal, we all worry about a whole host of things every day – jobs, relationships, money, Donald Trump being president of the United States. But *anxiety* as a disorder is a different beast. And while I'm happy to see it talked about more with less embarrassment, sometimes I think the term has been diluted somewhat. It's not a competition – if someone says they have anxious thoughts then you must respect that and listen to them, but I also think that the word is thrown around too freely at times. There is a sliding scale, for sure, but I suspect that if someone told you they were anxious, you might assume they just had a tendency to worry too much. In a bid to be more honest and less ashamed about my mad panic, I tell people more and more about what goes on with my anxiety – the past terrors and the remaining vestiges. But maybe I'm not blunt enough, because often I've told people and had a nod, a gesture of understanding, or sometimes just no reaction at all. It always amazes me, because I think if most people sat in my brain for a bit, they'd be shocked at how weird and intolerable it can get. The real release is talking to other people affected by it. A friend once called me to tell me that she'd decided that her neighbours might be out to get her. The anxiety behind this vague and weird thought was complex and impressive, but I *got* it. Because we both have weird and scary thoughts, we were able to fully spill all our irrational obsessions without the fear of being judged.

I guess what I'm saying is that anxiety is complex, messy and dark. It's not just panic attacks or a fear of crowded places – horrible things which are easy to understand by a general audience – but relentless obsessions, terrible thoughts, exhausting compulsions, physical malaise and deep sadness as a result. I think it's important, as we make strides to talk about mental illness, that we also make sure we know how grim and plain weird it can be. Progress and acceptance are not only achieved by being able to talk in general terms about mental health, or by highlighting stories of recovery – true understanding means bluntly talking about the hopelessness, the fear and the ugliness of it all too. The writer Hannah Jane Parkinson has written about her life with bipolar disorder so honestly that it helps you to see the reality of her illness. She does this without any hushed tones, or half-measures. 'There was the time I was sectioned and spent 22 hours in a "mental health suite" (read: a small, airless room with two chairs in it) waiting for a bed on an inpatient psychiatric ward (one was eventually found out of borough). There was being released from hospital after sectioning, therapy abruptly stopped, and having no continuing mental healthcare in place.'[20]

Anxiety doesn't go away, it controls your life. It stays with you at parties, at work, when you're with your loved ones on holiday, when you're safe in your bed. It affects your day-to-day life in a way that normal worries don't. If you're worrying about a job interview, those nerves tend to go away after the meeting is over. An anxious person will have worries that will likely mushroom. The interview could go perfectly well but the worries will remain, expand, mutate. They've got a hold of you and the grip is vice-like. Mixed anxiety and depression are the most common mental disorders in the UK – as many as 7.8 per cent of people meet the criteria for diagnosis.[21]

People worried about a specific issue might well experience deep distress, but people with anxiety will likely feel a vague sense of fear and nervousness *all* the time. Imagine they are successful in the job interview: while people without anxiety might have reasonable worries about how their first day in a new role might go – getting on with their new colleagues, or whether they will be up to the challenges a new job brings – people with anxiety will worry about a whole host of things that might not seem proportionate or rational. How will they cope travelling to work? How will they will handle a new routine? Will they fall over in front of their new colleagues? Could they get fired on their first day? What if they have a panic attack in the office? What if there's a fire and no clear exits? What if their dog dies while they're out? (I've had that fear before many times.)

When I started secondary school, I remember having the usual worries about the first day – making friends, finding the lessons too hard, fitting in. But within days of starting, I felt overwhelmed by them. I'd lie in bed worrying about the journey to school, being late, not knowing anyone, and whether I'd see my parents again (I told you anxiety can mushroom). I cried every single day that year, desperate not to go to the place which made me feel so scared and sad. I could not shake it off, and it didn't get better as time passed. Instead, my worries just mutated, latched onto new things, spread their roots through my mind. That was my first long period of anxiety, and it was the most distressing, because I was just eleven, and I didn't know what the hell was happening to me. A dear friend I made when I was thirteen told me that she used to tell her mum about 'the sad girl' in her year. That was me. What a nickname to have . . .

There are important physical differences too. While worry might make your stomach churn or give you sweaty palms, these symptoms will likely go away when a stressful situation passes. For a person with anxiety, the physical symptoms are legion. I mean it. There are hundreds of ways anxiety can impact on your body – chest pain, dizziness, headaches – and stranger ones. For me, I get a twitch in one eye, jumpy legs, ringing ears and a boiling-hot face. That's also a great description for a dating profile; feel free to use it.

At school, I often felt nauseated beyond belief. I'd get headaches, and feel dizzy, and I'd find it harder and harder to breathe. I constantly thought I had a problem that the GP could sort out, I begged for days off school. With the number of physical symptoms anxiety can bring on, it's no wonder people often worry that they are seriously ill. I said earlier that anxiety is a slippery thing. Sneaky, you might say. It can mimic other illnesses incredibly well. Health fears can become all-consuming – the first time people experience panic attacks, the most common assumption is that they are having a heart attack or a stroke. Later it can be a worry about brain tumours, MS, Parkinson's disease. The list goes on. And health anxiety isn't merely harmless worry. One study in Norway showed that people with such fears had a 73 per cent higher chance of developing heart disease over ten years than people who didn't have anxiety. [22] Lucky us, huh?

Anxiety and worry are different beasts. It's important to stress this, because if we want to understand mental health better while also reducing stigma, we must also understand how serious anxiety is. Just as depression is not just 'feeling sad', and postnatal depression is not simply the 'baby blues', anxiety is not just nerves. It's also really, really common. While the mental health stat most commonly heard is that one in four of us will suffer with mental-health problems in our life, those problems can sound pretty vague – many people probably don't know that anxiety and depression are the most common mental illnesses experienced.

So while there *are* other reasons a person might experience all-consuming worries, anxiety is the main factor in several mental health conditions. Before I bang on about what these are, let's state the obvious. I am not a mental-health expert and if you are worried that you might suffer from any of these disorders GO TO YOUR DOCTOR. Also the charity Mind is brilliant for advice and education – visit their website immediately. As the actress Carrie Fisher said of her bipolar: 'The only lesson for me, or for anybody, is that you have to get help. It's not a neat illness. It doesn't go away.'[23]

So without further ado, here are some of the most common anxiety disorders[24] (world's bleakest drumroll, please):

- Obsessive-compulsive disorder (OCD)
- Panic disorder
- Phobias – such as agoraphobia or claustrophobia
- Social anxiety disorder (social phobia)

- Post-traumatic stress disorder (PTSD)
- Generalised anxiety disorder (GAD)

Gather round while we talk a bit about them!

## OCD

It's important for me to start by saying that OCD is NOT ABOUT TIDYING YOUR CUPBOARDS. If I have to hear one more person airily tell me that they are really OCD about which direction their towels line up in, I will personally go over to their house and fold all their towels into horribly elaborate swan sculptures like they do in fancy hotels.

Despite the common misuse, OCD is a thoroughly nasty affliction, from which 1.2 people out of every 100 in the UK are thought to suffer.[25] It presents itself mainly in two ways: obsessions and compulsions. Both involve intrusive, unwelcome and terrifying thoughts. These are not simply the weird ideas your mind entertains at 2 a.m. on a Sunday night where you suddenly think about your parents doing it and hate your brain for traumatising you (though you do have my sympathy). No, these intrusive thoughts 'stick' in your head. One ordinary Tuesday afternoon you might suddenly imagine killing your child, or jumping in front of a train, but instead of chalking that odd idea up to a funny mind tic, you fixate on it. You are filled with panic and revulsion that you could think such a terrible thing – are you a murderer? Do you want to kill your baby? The terror consumes you, and the thought takes hold ever more firmly. In some instances, you ruminate, falling into ever more tangled thought patterns to try and 'neutralise' the thought. Try arguing with your exhausted and panicked brain about whether or not you might be a paedophile for

twelve hours straight and then tell me if you think your need
to line up shoes neatly is a bit OCD.

In *Mad Girl*, her memoir about mental illness, the writer
Bryony Gordon describes how these obsessions took hold in
painful detail. A fear of germs meant that 'I was so scared of
blood on my hands that I began to wash my hands as much
as possible, the irony being that they soon began to crack and
bleed.'[26] Later, she began to think she might have murdered
someone. That's how far the brain can travel with OCD. I
once drove around a roundabout several times thinking I'd
run someone over. There was nobody there. My brain still
wasn't convinced.

If you're not falling down a mental rabbit hole to try and
stop the horrible thoughts, then you might be acting out
compulsions. This pattern might go something like this: you
imagine your family dying in a horrible accident. You panic
about this horrible thought, and desperately need to figure
out a way to stop it. So your mind makes bargains with itself.
Just turn that light switch on and off twenty-five times when
you enter the room and they won't die. But don't forget! Oh
you think you missed a go? Well, do it five extra times to
be completely sure. And maybe add in a back-up – just to be
sure. Wash your hands until they are raw and bleeding and
cracked. Something still not feeling right? Do it again – if
you fuck it up, your family might die. Aged nine, I worried
that my mum might die while she was out if I didn't turn off
the light switch correctly. And I didn't really know what
correctly looked like, only that I'd 'feel' it when it was. That
meant turning the light on and off for hours. Yes, it sounds
stupid, but I was nine and thought my mum would die. That's
not something you can argue with rationally when you have

OCD. That's the illness. That's the impossible mind maze that you find yourself in. There's a good reason it's called the doubting disease.

On a lighter note, I do appreciate a well-hung towel too.

For people who have OCD without physical compulsions, there is just a cycle of irrational thoughts which whirr around the brain. Maz (not his real name) is divorced, and his ex-wife has primary custody of their children. Maz told me that he's engulfed by relentless thoughts that his kids have come to serious harm. 'I have images of accidents, my kids crying, of close calls with cars or balconies or whatever the fuck.' He imagines that they have died if he can't get hold of his ex. He will start to physically panic, which just leads to more intrusive thoughts. Sometimes Maz will convince himself that the thoughts are premonitions, or have come true, and he'll rush over to check on the children. Relief is always fleeting, as reassurance can only go so far (I used to spend hours googling OCD to try and calm myself down, but it worked briefly, if at all, and would actually prompt new fears, because I was giving them credence). Even without compulsions, you are always trying to counterbalance the terrible thoughts, and this can cause exhaustion and immense distress. Maz feels like he becomes a shell of himself when he's in the grip of obsessive thoughts: 'I can barely express myself or breathe, the morning light and air hurts, and I become convinced nothing will end well.'

I know this distress. Sometimes the ruminations get so bad that your mind starts skipping – like an old vinyl player getting stuck. You're so mentally exhausted that you start repeating words, phrases and sayings in your mind. You can't work your way out of the loop, and you feel hopeless. This, in turn, provokes fear, and then physical symptoms, and then back to obsessive thoughts. Do I sound overdramatic? I assure you, if anything, I'm downplaying it slightly for space reasons.

## Panic disorder

This is characterised by panic attacks – an extreme distortion of the fight-or-flight response. What's that? The fight-or-flight response is a basic human reaction triggered when we feel a negative emotion like fear. Obviously, it's very normal to feel fear when you're in danger. This response evolved to let us react quickly in a threatening situation: to fight, or to run away. The adrenaline released in such a situation allows us to move faster, gives us strength and makes our reactions sharper – some think it's what allows amazing examples of strength in a crisis – e.g. a mother managing to lift a car off her trapped son. That phenomenon has a great name – 'hysterical strength'.

But panic attacks can happen when there is no actual danger near. They seem to be triggered by false alarms, and the adrenaline and cortisol produced then work against us, making us hyperventilate, feel dizzy and shake after the fear has passed. But the danger seems so real, it's hard to believe there's nothing to be afraid of. Cue more attacks.

Before I explain the wide-ranging symptoms of such horrible attacks, it might first be helpful to describe what it feels like to actually *have* one. The worst panic attack I ever had took place in Finchley, North London. I suppose it was as good a place as any. I was eighteen, driving my car across a main road in a terrible storm. The cars were queuing up and slowing down, and the torrential rain meant driving through what looked like a lake in the middle of the road. My heart was beating fast, and my skin suddenly felt freezing cold, but I was pouring sweat. As I inched towards the 'lake', my ears roared with white noise and I started to lose my vision. Spots and flashes flew before my eyes and I couldn't breathe. I mean it. I could not catch a breath. I was heaving and gasping but no air seemed to be getting into my lungs. Every part of my body was shaking and nothing felt real anymore. My legs and arms felt detached from my body, and I believed I would die, right there in that car, crossing that stormy road. I didn't, of course. I got across. I pulled over. I shook uncontrollably for about twenty minutes, cried a lot and went home. You can bet I avoided that crossing for years.

Eleanor Morgan, the writer of *Anxiety for Beginners*, describes the first time she ever had a panic attack even more viscerally. Because it's the first one which is the most terrifying. The one where you feel you're dying for real. Later on you might know you're not, even though your body insists you're wrong. But that first one. Hoo boy. Morgan was at school, and ran to the loo, thinking she was going to vomit. But instead the cubicle started to move around her, and the walls felt 'like putty'.

'Nothing made sense to any one of my senses . . . what else, if not death, could be the end point of such physical and mental free fall?'[27]

Like Eleanor's, Beth's panic attacks started as a teenager. She told me that the symptoms terrified her, because they felt like a physical illness, as they do for so many initially. 'For a long time people definitely didn't believe what I was saying when I tried to explain how I felt. When it first started all the symptoms matched up with those of a stroke, my arms would become ridiculously heavy, I'd get numbness and tingles over my body, my eyesight would go, my body just felt like it was shutting down and it was terrifying. My legs turn to jelly, I shake, I get very cold, my stomach drops, I get dizzy. It can genuinely knock me out for a day after, which is great fun. I tense up so badly when it starts, [that] I just cause more issues for myself when it calms down. I hate not being in control, so trying to repress it is how I deal with it. It's never worked.'

Catherine's panic attacks also started at school – more particularly, at a stressful point in life – her GCSE exams. As is common, they were initially intensely physical. 'When I was sixteen and didn't understand that I had anxiety or that I was experiencing panic attacks, my symptoms were very physical – pounding chest, weak legs, blurry vision, knotted stomach, hyperventilating etc.,' Catherine told me. 'As I educated myself on the symptoms and the fight-or-flight response, my physical responses subsided and my symptoms became a lot more mental. My panic attacks now will manifest in a tense feeling and slight blurry vision and are now mostly uncontrollable, with fast thoughts racing around my head and feelings of detachment.'

Panic disorder means having several of these episodes a day – and they can last up to twenty minutes, and even longer attacks have been recorded. Imagine the fear just one panic attack can produce. Shaking, difficulty breathing, nausea, chest pain, fear of dying. The slump afterwards when the adrenaline leaves you. Then imagine how far you'd go out of your way to avoid another one. Just as I did in the car, people with panic disorder will often avoid a place where they've had an attack. This can limit your 'safe' places scarily fast. While it might feel like you're doing the sensible thing in not ushering in an attack, you're actually reinforcing the fear – giving it legitimacy. A person with panic disorder lives in fear of an attack, but will also have more general fears – meaning there is no real safe space for them at all.

Catherine has identified what brings on her attacks, and although everyone is different, I recognised a lot of my own triggers in what she said: 'Feeling out of control or not feeling as if I know enough about something. For example: going into town without having a plan of how I will be getting home, being spontaneous about plans, or going into a university class/exam unprepared.

'My second theme seems to be health related – I can get panic attacks related to doing things that could make my health worse, such as side effects of antibiotics or thinking I might be having allergic reactions to something. I also sometimes panic about the fear of passing out. If I'm very hungry, or I work out too hard, I can have a panic attack about the fear of passing out.'

While still having panic attacks, Catherine has done something I didn't do at her age: seeking help early. She has signed up for CBT sessions and also uses coping strategies when she senses that she might be about to have an attack:

'In the moment of panic my usual coping strategy is deep breathing, sipping water and mentally telling myself "there is no threat, everything is fine, and to be calm." I may remove myself from the situation if my panic is incredibly bad but usually I make myself stay, ride it out and show myself that what I'm panicking about isn't going to harm me. In terms of prevention I mostly use lifestyle – I get enough sleep, eat well, take vitamins, go for walks – generally just keep myself healthy and stress free. If I'm having an anxious time I can

recognise when I'm pushing myself too far and when to take
time to myself.'

**Phobias**

Almost everyone has a fear of something strange. The NHS
estimates 10 million people in the UK have some kind of
phobia.[28] My mum hates rats. For years, she wouldn't even
allow the word to be spoken in front of her. We had to say
'big mice'. My mother is incredibly strong, smart and fearless.
But I have seen her turn into a screeching mess when
confronted with 'big mice'. A country walk a few years ago
turned into a farce when we spied one twenty metres ahead
of us. 'TELL IT TO GO AWAY!' she yelled repeatedly as she
clutched my arm. Unhelpfully, I laughed uncontrollably at
this request. I am not a kind daughter. She can write her own
book about this.

But phobias can be life-changing. My mother rarely comes
into contact with rats. Other people are not so lucky with
their fears – and it can be incredibly distressing when you
sense danger – whether or not the danger is real.

Phobias usually fall into one of two categories – specific
phobias and complex ones. My mother has a specific phobia.
Animals are common, as are heights, blood, vomit and flying.
If you have a fear of something specific you'll normally go
out of your way to avoid it. If your phobia is massive spiders
and you don't live in Australia you might not find this too
restrictive but when it's something you can't always avoid,
you can find your world shrinks. I developed a fear of flying
aged eighteen. Having previously been fine on planes, I
suddenly could not get on a flight. I was terrified. I missed
fun family holidays, friends going on adventures, and work

trips. I occasionally took dreary train trips and pretended it was a fun way to travel, but I felt absurd and immobilised. Just the thought of a plane journey would have me shaking, and I felt so restricted by it.

Complex phobias are even harder to overcome. This term usually refers to agoraphobia and social phobia. Agoraphobia is widely assumed to be a fear of wide open spaces (a desert? the surface of the moon?) but is more likely to mean anxiety about how to get out of somewhere without panicking or where help is not obvious. Anxious people are often looking for the literal or metaphorical emergency exit. This might mean you feel overwhelmed on the Tube, or in a busy supermarket. Again, this can mean a person with agoraphobia might limit the places they go to. In the worst case, this might mean becoming housebound – the only place a person might feel truly safe. Agoraphobia often comes on after a bad experience – being stuck in a lift, or after having had an accident. Professor Kevin Gournay, an expert in the condition, estimates around 1 per cent of the UK population is affected by severe agoraphobia.[29]

Maybe this sounds like claustrophobia to you – the difference is small, but important. Claustrophobia is the extreme fear of confined or closed off spaces. With agoraphobia, you have a fear of any place that might make an easy escape difficult, leading to a panic attack or extreme anxiety.

**Social anxiety disorder**

Social anxiety disorder is also called social phobia. Just as depression is not feeling a bit sad, social anxiety does not mean being a bit shy at the office Christmas party. It's a crippling condition which can include fears of meeting new people, speaking in public, worrying you've embarrassed yourself in public, and having panic attacks in situations where you're forced to interact with people. People with social anxiety experience a lower quality of life than those unaffected, an increase in alcohol and drug abuse and a risk of suicide. In the UK, about five in every hundred people are thought to have some degree of social anxiety and it affects women more than men.[30] Perhaps unsurprisingly, it tends to develop in a person's teenage years and is unlikely to improve without help.

Ruchira told me that she's had fears about how others perceive her for as long as she can remember. Although it was uncomfortable, it wasn't until university that the anxiety element reared its head properly. 'I would excuse myself from seminars and just hyperventilate in the toilets without being able to return without the same panic happening. This was what I would call the flare-up – before this my anxiety had hindered me in smaller ways such as nervousness in crowds, fear of being looked at, attending events – things I never realised were different or I didn't have to feel.'

Ruchira explained that she never thought of herself as someone who would face such an issue – but then, who does? 'I'm a really outgoing confident person. I had the best time going out and meeting new people [before] so the idea I had social anxiety baffled me. I think social anxiety comes in different forms for so many people, and mine was all about how I'm weighed up in career settings or by my looks. "Being taken seriously" was a big anxiety, as I'd built an assumption that my young-looking face meant I had to make up for it or counteract people's thoughts before they got to know me.'

Eventually, her anxiety hit such high levels that she sought help, but it took a while. 'This came at a time of me rarely leaving the house and hitting the lowest state first. CBT made me realise [that] much of this stemmed from a fear of dying or fainting in front of everyone who I imagined would judge me. This mixture of panic and social anxiety – which had grown unchecked for years – had become something that meant I couldn't walk in crowds, get on the Tube, order food or anything without bursting into a panic attack. CBT really helped – along with a citalopram [SSRI] prescription.'

So you see – social anxiety – not just shyness at all.

## Post-traumatic stress disorder (PTSD)

The *Diagnostic and Statistical Manual of Mental Disorders* (*DSM*) provides definitions of mental-health problems. It explains that PTSD triggers include exposure to actual or threatened death, serious injury or sexual violation. The trauma, regardless of trigger, causes significant distress or impairment to a person's social interactions, and their ability to work or function in other normal ways.

PTSD is most commonly understood to be seen in soldiers after combat – recorded throughout history during the American Civil War as 'heart shock', in the First World War as 'shellshock', and then in the Second World War as 'combat fatigue'.[31] But it's now known to affect those who have experienced sexual assault, violence and accidents, traumatic childbirth and disasters. Symptoms of PTSD include repeated thoughts of the assault or incident, nightmares, avoiding thoughts and situations related to the trigger; feeling unsafe, panic attacks, and difficulty sleeping and concentrating. According to NHS figures, PTSD is estimated to affect about one in every three people who have a traumatic experience, though it's not known exactly why some people are affected and others aren't.[32]

Sufferers don't just experience the trigger clearly, they can also relive the experience through flashbacks, where a word, smell or noise might make a person think the trauma they endured is happening again. Understandably, those with PTSD will often go out of their way to avoid anything that might provoke a flashback – changing their routines or restricting their movements. They will be hyper-vigilant, watching for danger at every turn. This can provoke huge anxiety because of the constant mental pressure to be alert.

Further types of PTSD have since been defined, to better reflect the different experiences of it. They include:

*Delayed-onset PTSD*. If your symptoms emerge more than six months after experiencing trauma, this could be described as 'delayed PTSD' or 'delayed-onset PTSD'.

*Complex PTSD*. This encompasses chronic and prolonged trauma or abuse. For example, if a person suffered from years of domestic violence, they might be said to have 'complex PTSD'.

As with all mental-health problems, sufferers can live with the symptoms for years before diagnosis. Nicola was diagnosed with PTSD as an adult, having been sexually abused by her father as a young teenager. She only sank into a depression after leaving her job in the RAF and returning to civilian life. Even though she was offered counselling, Nicola found it hard to talk about what had happened to her, partly because a therapist wouldn't 'know what it is like to experience it'.

A fear of stigma is common in people who suffer with PTSD. For those who've been sexually abused like Nicola, victim-blaming attitudes and a fear of not being believed can prevent people from seeking help as early as possible. This is compounded by feelings of shame and guilt that many with PTSD experience.

I've been lucky not to experience this awful disorder in any real sense, though I am familiar with hyper-vigilance. After being stalked a few years ago, I was advised by the counselling service provided by Victim Support that I might experience some symptoms of PTSD. I didn't think I was likely to, given that my troubles weren't as serious as I thought those suffering from the disorder face, but I certainly did feel hyper-vigilant – looking for and sensing danger everywhere. I repeatedly checked under the bed, locked and unlocked doors, tested my alarm and felt on edge – prone to fright at every noise and movement. I was also just feeling highly anxious, with all my usual symptoms dialled up to eleven. As with all anxiety illnesses, it can therefore be hard to decipher which one you are experiencing. If PTSD seems like it might be something you're suffering from, there are many resources available to you – starting with your own GP; but also including the mental health charity Mind, Combat Stress (for veterans' mental health), the Royal College of Psychiatrists, and PTSD UK. Links are to be found at the back of the book.

## Generalised anxiety disorder (GAD)

Hello old friend! Generalised anxiety disorder is sort of exactly what it sounds like – a free-floating but excessive level of worry which can't be shrugged off. Nearly six people out of 100 are thought to suffer from generalised anxiety disorder in this country, [33] and *DSM-5* (the fifth edition of the most popular diagnostic system for mental disorders in the US) says the

period of time a person suffers for before diagnosis is important – it puts it at at least six months, to highlight the
difference between those with worries based on something
specific in life, and those for whom worries will not pass no
matter what happens. This kind of anxiety means you worry
even when there's nothing actually wrong, or in a way that's
disproportionate to any actual risk. When you get on top of
one worry, another will pop up – and your mind always races
to the worst possible scenario in each case.

These worries will nearly always have a physical effect too.
You may 'feel' a sense of doom, have headaches, suffer from
insomnia or feel tired or rundown all the time. Other fun
results of GAD that I've experienced include a terrible short-
term memory; difficulty concentrating on anything; and a
massive sense of irritation, directed at myself and others. There
are countless other symptoms, which I still sometimes look
up on dubious medical sites as a special treat (I'm kidding: I
do it to tick off any weird pains I have). The disorder affects
women more than men, and it's a contributing factor in some
cases of depression too, hastening the need for treatment.

Much is written about stress in the modern world. The
Office for National Statistics says an estimated 137.3 million
working days were lost due to sickness or injury in the UK in
2016, and that a third of those days were lost to mental-health
issues.[34] We're constantly told that our lives are full of worry
– about money, work, family and relationships. These very real
issues can make the most relaxed person feel anxious. GAD
means you might worry *frantically* about these issues – as well
as a whole host of other ones which seem to tack on to the
initial one. I can easily spend hours worrying about money,
which seems like a rational focus, but my mind will immedi-

ately take me to a place where I'm stranded, bankrupt and chased by debtors. On top of that, I'll suddenly feel besieged by anxiety about illness, about whether I might have offended someone at work, about whether I remembered to blow out a forgotten candle, or maybe I'll start thinking I'm getting a serious illness. One worry ushers in another, and another, until your mind is swarming with them and you feel almost despairing. It's a tangled web that happens in warp speed – you don't know where to begin trying to tackle the mess.

David suffers with GAD, having lived with anxiety for as long as he can remember. 'When it's at its worst, it manifests itself in both physical and emotional ways. Physically, I always feel tense, have sweaty palms, am quite restless and unable to concentrate for long periods. If something is on my mind I get full-blown stomach aches, palpitations, sweating. Mentally and emotionally it manifests itself in constant worrying, racing thoughts – the inability to rationalise things or live with uncertainty. For instance, if I am unsure of how a meeting at work might go, I will obsess about it all day, and be unable to focus on anything else until it is resolved. I have phobias of certain things – flying, food poisoning/general health problems. It's exhausting all round, really.'

Exhausting, because your whole body is trying to expend excess adrenaline. The adrenaline that comes with GAD is extraordinary. My default position is lying down in bed, snoozing away. But at my most anxious, I have the energy of a young gazelle. I could do star jumps for hours if I wasn't so busy feeling like shit and biting off the skin around my nails while I tap my feet and fail to concentrate on anything for more than thirty seconds. It comes in like a violent wave to the shore, knocking over anything in its wake, and shocking you with its force. You wake up to it rushing into your belly, pushing up into your throat, telling you that danger is near. Adrenaline – great in a real crisis, terrible when there's nothing to worry about. It feels way too real to be ignored, so you don't. Something must be wrong. In a real crisis, adrenaline (and its ugly sisters norepinephrine and cortisol) might help you pull a child from a burning building with Herculean effort. With anxiety, you just feel physically ill – a sweaty, shaky, nauseous bundle of nerves. This contributes to a feedback loop – you feel physically full of fear; and this adrenaline might cause a panic attack. After that has subsided, you look for reasons as to why it happened – leading to ruminations and obsessive thoughts searching for a legitimate cause. You spend a lot of time fearing another episode of panic and that leads to extra adrenaline . . . and on and on.

The other symptom of GAD that I always find overpowering is the feeling of impending DOOM it can bring. I remember visiting a local supermarket with my mother several years ago, when I suddenly felt as though the world was about to end. The colours in the shop felt all wrong, and everyone around me looked sinister and unfriendly. I could feel my emotions plummeting, as though a dementor from *Harry Potter* had sucked all of the joy out of my body. From nowhere, I felt utter dread, as all the while people were just buying their dinner. The doom sensation is incredibly scary – you feel like there *must* be a reason for it – just as with adrenaline rushes, it's hard to shake it off and chalk it up to anxiety when every part of you is telling you that danger is approaching.

This feeling of doom is not unique to me or my fellow sufferers in the twenty-first century. In 1773, London physician George Cheyne wrote *The English Malady*, a book in which he addressed his own anxiety, describing his 'fright, dread and terror'.[35] He might not have experienced it in his local Sainsbury's, but the feelings are the same.

I've described some of the anxiety illnesses most commonly seen. But maybe you don't get the doom, or the panic attacks, or the weird eye-twitching. That doesn't mean you don't have anxiety, or that your experience is abnormal. I could write a book on all the various symptoms alone, or a PhD which would entirely consist of the mad thoughts and neuroses that I've had in my life. Nobody would read it though, probably not even me. I say this to reassure you that even if none of this sounds like you, it doesn't mean that your anxiety is less awful or somehow not as life-affecting as anybody else's. Mental health is not a Top Trumps game (this probably dates me horribly), and if anxiety has given me anything positive, it's taught me to be more empathetic with others who struggle in life. We all have bad brain stuff. Don't minimise your stuff, or compare it with other people's. Having a loving family or a good job doesn't mean you have to stay quiet when you're struggling with mental-health problems – however small you think they are. You know better than anyone else whether something in your brain feels wrong – and if it does, seek help. Anxiety disorders usually get worse without intervention – whatever that ends up meaning for you. The things that have worked for me have been therapy, drugs and running. Your version of help might be different, but do make a serious effort to seek it out. It'll be the best thing you can ever do for yourself, and for those who love you.

Anxiety is nothing new. Ancient Latin and Greek litera-
ture repeatedly references fear and worry. In the seventeenth
century, the Oxford scholar Robert Burton described anxiety
in his book *The Anatomy of Melancholy*, in which he wrote
'what cannot be cured, must be endured'[36] – a pretty good
saying even now. Panic attacks were referred to as 'pano-
phobias' in the eighteenth century, and we've all heard the
phrase 'attacks of the vapours'. In 1869, American doctor
George Miller Beard described neurasthenia – meaning
nervous weakness – as a condition that the middle class was
increasingly suffering from.[37] He believed that they were
overcome by the rapid advance of modern society. Come
talk to me about rapid advance now, Beard: just try to use
a parking meter without a phone, a credit card or a degree
in maths.

Sigmund Freud wrote that 'anxiety [is] a riddle whose
solution would be bound to throw a flood of light on our
whole mental existence.'[38] He spent a lot of time thinking
about this particular mental-health problem, and initially
thought that anxiety had something to do with the trauma
of being born. Later he suggested it was probably also about
the death instinct or some form of aggression operating within
ourselves. Above all, he thought it was connected to the helplessness of infants – who can't survive without the assistance
of other people, creating a trauma that sticks with us. Then
again, Freud came up with the Oedipal theory, so I'm shocked,
that like Philip Larkin, he didn't chalk anxiety up to your
mum and dad fucking you up.

But despite this wealth of material, anxiety as a stand-alone
mental illness was not recognised properly until the 1980
publication of *DSM-3*, which had a chapter on anxiety disor-

ders. [39] These included phobic disorders, social phobia, panic disorder, GAD, obsessive-compulsive disorder (OCD) and post-traumatic stress disorder (PTSD). Wahooo! We were recognised! It's nice to finally get some recognition . . . I'd like to thank my family, my friends and my dog.

This stand-alone diagnosis is important – no longer would anxiety be lumped in with other mental-health issues (though of course, many overlap). And that coincided with the introduction of treatments that might actually work. Thank God we now live in an age where medicine is not only effective but also has the added benefit of not being utterly punishing. Not for us the hideous 'have a bash' treatments that the mentally ill suffered through the ages – trepanning (having a hole drilled into your head to reduce pressure), lobotomy (which involved severing neural connections in the brain so as to relieve certain severe mental conditions), diathermia (using a current on the brain to jolt patients with psychosis), or being submerged in freezing water to treat women with hysteria. Hysterical women crop up a lot in history – from Hippocrates, who thought women's wombs wandered (what a band name), to English doctor Thomas Sydenham, who wrote that hysteria was a malady which nearly all women suffered from – 'there is rarely one who is wholly free from it.'[40] The Victorians were mad for trying to give women orgasms – whether or not they wanted them – to stop women being unhappy or angry, or maybe just not the perfect subservient wives that men expected. Between 1864 and 1889, entries at one asylum in Virginia recorded the reasons that patients were said to have become unwell. These included: laziness, egotism, disappointed love, 'female disease', imaginary female trouble, jealousy, religion, asthma, masturbation and 'bad habits'.[41] Worryingly vague, and although not given as the main reason for admission, they seem hard to disprove . . .

As an aside, if you want to read more about how women with mental-health problems have been treated over the years, read *Mad, Bad and Sad* by Lisa Appignanesi.[42] It's fascinating on the subject of how women are still much more often categorised as mentally unwell or 'unbalanced' than men.

The most effective treatment for anxiety is usually agreed to be talking therapy, which many credit Freud with bringing to the fore. His famous description of Josef Breuer's treatment of the patient Anna O. (later revealed to be Austrian Bertha Pappenheim, the founder of the League of Jewish Women) is widely regarded as the beginning of psychoanalysis. Guess what she was diagnosed with? Yup, hysteria.

Cognitive behavioural therapy (CBT) is now seen as one of the most effective types of treatment for anxiety disorders – and the one recommended by the NHS.[43] Developed in the 1960s by Aaron Beck, it's a form of therapy which involves re-examining your thought patterns and challenging negative behaviour. CBT is also recommended in the treatment of depression, schizophrenia and bipolar disorder and there is evidence it can help with chronic fatigue, anger issues and sleep problems. Having had therapists in the past who were very keen to start right back in my early childhood and work through my entire life in a bid to find the one key thing that made me anxious, I was relieved to try CBT and cut out much of this process. The first thing I was given was homework – a sheet of paper with boxes on it. In these, I had to write down my big irrational thoughts and what I thought would happen if the worst came true. Sometimes the sheets would look like this:

*Huge worry: What if I start hearing voices and believe aliens are trying to abduct me?*

*Likelihood: HIGH.*

*Conclusion: I'll have to live in an asylum and I'll never see my family again.*

The homework then required me to write down the worry again, and then to consider a more realistic conclusion:

*Huge worry: What if I start hearing voices and believe aliens are trying to abduct me?*

*Likelihood: Actually pretty low – in 2014, an estimated 0.7 per cent of the UK population were reported to show symptoms of psychosis disorder.* [44]

*Conclusion: While there is a slim chance that I might have a psychotic illness, there are many people who live full lives while coping with serious mental-health problems, and very few people end up in what I think of as 'asylums' anymore. There would be a plan of action and I would have great support in place.*

I was sceptical of such a method – I'd been dealing with catastrophic worries for years; it felt too simplistic to merely write down my worries and try and reframe them. But what do you know? It started to work. I'd write these alternative conclusions and quickly forget them. Later on, when inevitably another new and SCARIER worry cropped up, I'd do my normal freak-out and start falling down the rabbit hole of catastrophe. But then something would stop me – I'd remember the worksheet and ask myself if I could see a different outcome, whether maybe I had a choice in how far I chose to take the thought. I still do this in my head from time to time – when I feel my thoughts racing and have to rein them in.

CBT has worked for me, and for many others who have been lucky enough to receive this treatment. But current NHS waiting list times often mean that medication is offered first.[45] In the course of writing this book, so many people I spoke to were still on the waiting list to have a limited number of CBT sessions, and would take medication as they waited for talking therapy. The is medication most commonly prescribed for anxiety disorders is selective serotonin reuptake inhibitors (SSRIs), which are thought to increase the levels of the chemical serotonin in your brain. After carrying a message between nerve cells in the brain, serotonin is usually reabsorbed by the cells. SSRIs work by blocking this absorption, meaning more serotonin is available to pass further messages between nearby nerve cells. You might also be offered serotonin–noradrenaline reuptake inhibitors (SNRIs), which increase both chemicals, or benzodiazepines, which have a sedative effect and can't be used for a long period of time because they're addictive. Speaking personally, they're bloody amazing for a short window where you're finding it hard to get through the day. But be aware that the doctor will probably not give you more than two weeks' worth, for good reason. Especially if you go in wild-eyed, praising them and loudly insisting you must have more. Not my subtlest move.

Whatever meds you're prescribed, you'll start on a low dose, and be monitored by your GP to see whether you need a higher dose, and to check your side effects. Don't expect relief immediately; usually these drugs don't become fully effective for 2–4 weeks, which I know can feel interminable, but don't stop taking them, or give up hope.

As with so much to do with mental illness, taking drugs for mental-health problems still comes with a huge stigma attached. This is in part because some who have not had cause to take them find it hard to understand why other people do. It's also to do with ignorance, or a lack of education around what the meds actually *do*. Headlines in some sections of the media don't help, to put it mildly. A NATION HOOKED ON HAPPY PILLS yelled the *Daily Mail* at the end of 2017[46] – the implication being that those of us who take antidepressants do so for an easy fix, or for a high that doesn't actually exist.

So, for clarity: does taking antidepressants mean that you're crazy? (No.) Do they mean you're dangerous? (No.) Don't they make you a robot unable to feel emotions? (Hahaha. NO.) But yet still we feel shame or hesitancy in telling those we love about them. A 2011 study showed that one in three women in the UK will take antidepressants in their lifetime, and yet 18 per cent won't tell their families and one in ten won't tell their partner. [47] I hesitated to tell my partner that I took medication, worried he'd think less of me. Ridiculous, really. And he didn't. At all.

I shouldn't need to argue why it's so important not to judge someone for taking medication when they're struggling. I'd love it if we lived in a world where taking SSRIs was just like taking paracetamol for a headache. But we're not there yet. I've been taking them on and off for years now, but I didn't tell anyone about them for fear of looking like I was abnormal. I didn't know anyone that took them and I didn't want to be any different. Except I did. I knew tons. When I finally told people (gradually, cautiously) so many of my friends and family said that they'd had cause to use them at some point in their lives too. Some for a few months, some for a few years. Some were adamant they'd never come off them. A few people were surprised I was being open about it, and urged me not to disclose it to employers, showing that the stigma is *real*.

I've not come to any fixed conclusion about how long I'll continue to take them. But I do know that, personally, they dug me out of the pits of despair and took me back to a place where I could think about something other than death and destruction. They didn't flatten my emotions, rather, they let me feel something other than utter misery. They gave me the chance to start figuring out what would help me be actually happy. Because I'm sorry to disappoint but they don't make you happy – no matter what fear-mongering headline might scream about mind-altering drugs. They just give you a chance to not be so fucking sad. And they don't work for everyone, and they can come with some pretty serious side effects. I get night sweats (gross and fun to explain to a new partner), and you might feel nausea; or dizziness; or lose interest in sex, but not always, and you have to decide for yourself how much you can put up with. Either way, don't be scared off medication by people who freely judge because they've never experienced the sadness and worry that others have. Lucky them, but you do you.

If you need further reassurance, a 2018 study (published in the *Lancet*) which looked at the efficacy of twenty-one antidepressants found that all the drugs tested were more effective than a placebo in adults with major depressive disorder[48] – though sadly the data can't show which drug would be most likely to work best for any individual. The six-year study was hailed by many experts, who heralded the results as a blow to the lingering stigma that still surrounds medication for anxiety and depression.

For all the talking therapy and medication I was lucky enough to be given, however, I was never able to completely get myself on an even keel. The drugs took me out of doom, the talking reassured me that I could keep my thoughts in check better, but I always felt like both were only getting me so far. It was as if I was always tentatively standing on the top of a hill, while everyone skied past me and beckoned me down (I've never skied, it looks completely terrifying). And that's fine – nothing is a miracle cure and you can't expect total relief from one remedy. I'm glad I was able to get help from both, and I'm still grateful that they got me to a stage where I could find more things that helped. Things that might help me get to be really happy and not in a place where I was just 'managing'.

It's not that managing is a terrible place to be, but it can be stultifying. When you get there, it feels amazing – as though you've jumped a massive hurdle. But then you find that there are other hurdles in the distance, and it's frustrating when you want to tackle them too. That's another little annoyance that mental-health problems are likely to throw up – however far you've got with your recovery or management, there are always other levels to tackle, new fears to confront. The journey is never completely over – no final, happy end to the worries you'll face. It's a long and sometimes slow process, but once you're on board, you realise how much better it is to be taking it than the alternative. That doesn't mean that you won't get disheartened, but remember how far you've come already. And at the risk of sounding like a motivational coach, your progress is your own. When I realised I could go on the Tube without fainting for the first time in sixteen years, I was prouder than a stage-school parent at a recital. The feeling was indescribable, and I carry that memory with me when I feel like I'm not as brave or as competent as those around me. Small steps.

# 3K – SUFFER THE LITTLE CHILDREN

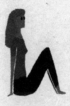

Today I ran for ten minutes without checking my timer. This is a first — usually I can't help but see what I've managed (or worse, how little I've done). Ten minutes seems like a real milestone — a concrete achievement that I can't brush off. Ten minutes in a straight line, away from the sanctuary of my house. As usual, my mind protested initially — kicking off with questions and 'what ifs' — trying to send me scurrying for home. But by minute five, I wasn't listening. I was looking out for the schoolkids huddled in groups eating fried chicken outside the school gates, and the women with enormous buggies laden with children and shopping which force me into the road. I ran away from the main road and pushed myself up a hill. My arms seemed to be powering my body, pumping naturally from side to side as I raised myself onto the balls of my feet and sped up. I felt joy as I went, as if I was used to doing this every day, as if my limbs were just doing what they loved. Every part of my body seemed in sync for the first time, as though I was a natural runner and not a painful amateur. I managed eighteen minutes and discovered physical exhilaration.

\* \* \*

Childhood is, hopefully, a time when you learn and explore, free from the certain burdens of adulthood. It's also usually the time when you do the most exercise, though a 2013 study by University College London found that British children don't do nearly enough.[49] And it's important that they do loads. The World Health Organisation recommends that children aged 5–17 have at least an hour of physical activity a day, to strengthen the heart and bones, increase mobility, and maintain a healthy weight. A 2017 study in Norway went further, showing that moderate to vigorous exercise in 6–8 -year-olds meant they were less likely to show symptoms of major depressive disorder two years later.[50] Inevitably, the study also showed that the older children got, the less physical activity they took each day. Maybe that's why you can now get a Fitbit which is designed specifically for children – encouraging them to take 250 steps every hour. Though I suspect that it wouldn't have worked on a kid like me.

In my childhood, I definitely didn't do the requisite hour, I didn't even do fifteen minutes a day. I determinedly did as little as I could get away with. Very early on, I realised that the chubby kid with little team spirit would probably not be picked for football or relay races. A juvenile sense of pride and a healthy dose of self-consciousness meant that I resolved not to try at all. I sat out years of tugs of war, rounders, bleep tests, swim groups and tennis. I would not run for a bus. I didn't even play kiss chase (though I don't think the boys were lining up for the chance anyway, bastards). I regretted none of this until much later in my life.

Instead, I was mostly stationary. I did other things. I read, I painted, I discovered TV and I did a *lot* of eating. I didn't develop netball skills or win any relay races, I focused on honing my burgeoning anxiety problem. Obviously I didn't know I had an anxiety problem. I just cried uncontrollably when my mum went out, imagining terrible things would befall her out in the dangerous and scary world beyond our front gate. I felt sick more than most kids. I got frightened by things that weren't even scary – a surreal painting, a piece of music, a loud car. I didn't want to try new things. My chest hurt a lot. My stomach ached. I had bad dreams, and worried about the people I loved way too much for such a little kid.

While the NHS estimates that 300,000 young people have an anxiety disorder, only 2–5 per cent of kids under twelve will be affected.[51] I was one of them. Lucky me!

While I remember earlier examples of separation anxiety, my clearest memory of anxiety as a child came at age seven, when I attended a school party with my mum. My chest began to hurt as we queued up for the food stall. It hurt. I went quiet and held my neck, trying to breathe normally. I asked my mum if we could go home, but we'd only just got there and there wasn't anything obviously wrong with me – not anything I could adequately explain, at least. Eventually, we did leave early, because I wouldn't let up. Something felt strange and scary. Even aged seven, I knew that my house would provide the safety I wanted.

This small episode was to be a small taste of what was to come, even though it would be many years before I had any idea what was wrong with me.

Anxiety has been with me for as long as I can remember, but it's ebbed and flowed over the years. Just when I thought I'd got a handle on it, or banished it for good, it would rear its head as if in triumph, and bring with it new and more terrifying symptoms that would floor me.

At eleven, I went to secondary school and the change sent me into a tailspin. I cried every day, much like many other kids who hate moving to a new place and making new friends, but I didn't stop there. I developed OCD tics – swallowing whenever I had a bad or negative thought, blinking to neutralise fears about school, even more disgustingly, spitting – as if to rid bad feelings from my body as quickly as possible. I had no idea what this meant – I just knew I 'had' to do them. They absorbed me, I remember missing my bus stop in the mornings many times because I hadn't blinked in the correct way. There was no winning – the goalposts would shift all the time, my own mind coming up with new ways to try and trick me or catch me out. If it wasn't blinking, it was avoiding cracks in the pavement – small things that paralysed me. It feels silly to recall how flummoxed I would get by pavements, how I would have to retrace steps and start again if I did it 'wrong'.

These routines would take up hours of my time, partly in the doing and partly in the concealing – I was very adamant that those around me must not know. I also found myself disassociating for the first time – detaching from my surroundings when it all got too much. This remains my most terrifying anxiety symptom, and the one I can't totally shake off. Though it's believed that your brain dissociates during moments of high anxiety in an attempt to protect you, it only ever makes me feel much much worse, as though I'm drowning but my legs don't work when I try and frantically kick. The room, and everyone in it, begin to feel unreal. Colour gets too bright, sounds are jarring and it feels like I'm cocooned in bubble-wrap, unable to get back to reality. I first felt this at a bar mitzvah party, and it terrified me so much that I can't remember anything else about the night.

At worst, I've looked in the mirror at my own face and not recognised it to be me, and not just because I had terrible hair and bad skin that morning. It's a strange and fucking awful experience. I remember being ten, and going on holiday with a friend for the first time. I only managed one night, where everything and everyone looked strange and sinister and I thought I must been broken in some way (separation anxiety stuck with me for years – my poor parents must have been desperate for some time alone). When I'm stressed out, it still floods back. When I was trapped in a fug of anxiety and depression in my early twenties, disassociation made it feel as though the people around me were actors in a bad reality show – my adrenaline pumped, and my emotions were heightened, and this somehow managed to make loved ones seem like cardboard cutouts. I couldn't cut through to connect with them – everything felt fake and staged – like I was in the uncanny valley. (The uncanny-valley hypothesis is centred on humanoid objects which appear almost, but not exactly, like real human beings. They make us feel spooked and creeped out.)

I still think this is why I started to worry that I might be psychotic later in life. Human beings have an innate desire to connect to each other. We suffer when our bonds are broken – a romantic relationship severed, or a friendship which fades away. We need to feel close to others. But with disassociation, all of that goes. It's as if a glass wall is put up between you and those you love – blurring and distancing you. I used to look at my beloved family and see strangers. Nothing scared me more.

What else? Well, I would scratch and pick at my skin, until it bled and scarred, pull out hairs (a mild form of trichotillomania, where sufferers have an intense urge to pull their hair out and feel a strong sense of relief when they do, and more common in teenagers than adults), and I'd chew my lips until they bled. All fun scars to have as an adult. 'Why do you have scars all up your legs Bella?' 'Oh just because I pull and pluck my leg hair until I bleed when I feel like I'm losing control; who wants another drink?'

I didn't tell anyone about these symptoms, as terrifying as I found them to be. I was embarrassed, and scared that if I spoke about what was going on, bad things would happen. I still don't know exactly what these bad things were, but the threat of them felt very real to me as an unhappy eleven-year-old. I felt doom looming all the time. If I'd read Kafka as a weirdly precocious kid, I'd have nodded at his description of worry. 'The feeling of having in the middle of my body a ball of wool that quickly winds itself up, its innumerable threads pulling from the surface of my body to itself.'[52] (I didn't, obviously, I read Enid Blyton.)

These days, help is fortunately more easily available for children who exhibit the symptoms I did in my early years – charities like Young Minds offer excellent information and advice if you know a kid that needs it – but I've no doubt that many kids still suffer with scary thoughts and compulsions which they tell nobody about. As sympathetic as my parents were, I don't think any serious thought was given to whether I had mental-health problems. 'Bella gets nervous' was definitely a common refrain, but the assumption was very much that I would grow out of it. Perhaps if I'd told them that I was making increasingly complicated pacts with myself so that they wouldn't die, they might have worried more. But I didn't.

And anyway, I did grow out of it. For a bit. Awkward as

a little kid, I flourished in my teenage years, prioritising my social life over everything else. I felt like I fitted in for the first time in my short life – no odd tics, no detaching from the world around me, no sore chest, no worrying my mum would die if I forgot to blink the correct number of times. I hopped around London happily like all my friends, thinking my early years had been an unlucky blip.

I found friends and fun, and this meant that in many ways I was able to push my usual anxiety symptoms to the back of my mind – making me a luckier teenager than most. It's common knowledge that your adolescent years are, at best, tricky and at worst, unbearable. And that's not just because of the normal trials of puberty, which are bad enough on their own. Fifty per cent of mental illnesses in adult life start before the age of fifteen and 75 per cent have shown themselves by the age of eighteen. And mental-health problems in teens are thought to be on the rise: a study by the Department of Education in 2017 found that one in three teenage girls suffer from anxiety or depression – up 10 per cent in a decade. Neuropsychiatric conditions are the leading cause of disability in young people across the globe, and if they are left untreated at this crucial period in life, teenagers risk missing out on education and opportunity, and facing isolation and stigma. In other words, it's obviously crucial to tackle this stuff early, and it's becoming more and more obvious that exercise can play a big part in this. While the NHS recommends that 5–18-year-olds do sixty minutes of exercise each day for the physical benefits, the Royal College of Psychiatry emphasises the benefits of regular exercise for young minds too.

But I, like many others, didn't tackle my worries early enough – I was too busy suppressing them and working to pass as 'normal.' I skipped PE, sat still, unknowingly nurturing the seed of worry I'd contained for so long. So much progress has been made in the past few years to dismantle the stigma and shame of mental illness – I still marvel at the changes, even though there's always more that can be done. But even fifteen years ago, my only understanding of mental illness was of psychosis – and a dramatised, inaccurate version at that. We didn't learn about mental health at school, and nobody talked about it openly – except flippantly and with the certain knowledge that it would never affect us, only other people. Only that wasn't true – two close friends had psychotic episodes around this time. They popped up from time to time after treatment, but they were never the same boys as before. And we didn't understand what had happened, feeling as if it was best to gloss over it and move on. So I never thought I might be ill, or need help with my worries. And so, surely, they slowly crept back. It started with trouble breathing – maybe I had asthma (nope, panic attacks). Then I got headaches and worried I had a brain tumour (nope, see above). I felt ill and tired all the time. I fainted in a club, and took that to mean I was seriously sick.

The first onset of long-term mental-health problems usually shows up in adolescence, although treatment normally comes later. So I was bang on time. I didn't know what was going on, but I started to use my own methods (again) to tackle my symptoms, coming up with incredibly complex and ridiculous excuses to explain them away. I became the designated driver on nights out in case anything bad happened to the girls who were drinking (really it was because I was terrified of terrorist attacks and somehow thought having a car would help me). I no longer took the Tube and airily made jokes about how I didn't want to be treated worse than cattle (I would have panic attacks in confined spaces). I wouldn't drive on motorways in case I had a panic attack and crashed, but I got around this by offering to drive on other journeys. I stopped flying, though this was harder to explain – I had to admit I was scared and I hated telling the truth about it. If we went to a bar or club with no obvious exit I would immediately feel ill. I didn't know why, and it became a joke that I carried paracetamol and apple juice everywhere – as if they were my weapons and might help in any emergency somehow. I quickly lost the carefree attitude I'd assumed was mine forever.

I made friends and boyfriends leave cinemas and theatres if I felt boxed in. I cancelled on people constantly if I felt something was 'off' about the event, and yet still I didn't put two and two together to realise I had anxiety. My first boyfriend, poor man, had to put up with a lot of strange behaviour that I never understood myself, let alone could explain to him. I cried at a lot of dinners. I fled from a lot of dinners. The writer Scott Stossel nails it brilliantly in his memoir about living with anxiety: 'I've abandoned dates, walked out of exams, and had breakdowns in job interviews, on plane flights, train trips and car rides, and simply walking down the street.'[53] I lost friends because I couldn't articulate why I was so flaky. And even then, I'd figure it was a price worth paying 'to be safe'.

My coping skills were rubbish; but they got me by for a few years. I could still enjoy life up to a point; and I still felt pretty 'normal', just sick sometimes; and breathless a lot. I went to the GP too much, with various complaints, trying to tackle the symptoms without knowing the cause. If I had known what was wrong with me, I often wonder whether I'd have taken the steps we now know help to ease anxiety – breathing properly, mindfulness, taking exercise. Probably not. I was far too self-conscious to do anything that might seem weird or draw attention to myself. In terms of avoiding physical activity, I was not alone. Research by Sport England shows that at almost every age, women do less exercise than men.[54] The reasons why are complex, but feedback showed that sport is associated with natural talent, aggression, not being feminine, and being too competitive. Fear of being judged comes up again and again.

Bluntly, I didn't want to exercise because I thought people would laugh at me. I wasn't any good at group sports and I felt as though I'd look foolish if I tried. The boys' school up the road had acres of sports fields – football, cricket, rugby, track. They all seemed to be on the go every day of the week. But we were given half-hearted gym classes, where we threw balls around, or were made to climb an ancient, dusty pommel horse. By sixth form, the school made it clear we were on our own. We had walks around the local park, which I took to mean 'smoking in the bushes'. I was good at that PE class. The campaign 'This Girl Can' has worked hard to show women and girls that exercise is vital for wellbeing, and nothing to feel embarrassed about, but it's a hard stigma to crack, especially when girls have mixed PE lessons and have to worry about comments from boys, something one study showed was a main concern.

While this might not be given as the main reason for women's reluctance to exercise, I've always suspected sexism features strongly. Things are changing, but when I was growing up the boys were expected to play football and the girls were supposed to make daisy chains or do chalk drawings . . . or just sit quietly. Sadly, this doesn't seem to have changed radically. In 2016 sports journalist Anna Kessel wrote a book, *Eat, Sweat, Play*, encouraging girls to exercise. She describes actually seeing the differing expectations placed on boys and girls when it comes to sport – and neither tactic is encouraging. Chancing upon a football lesson for boys, she watches as the kids playing are neither encouraged nor praised, but chided when they failed. 'Many were half-hearted in their efforts, and their teacher barely acknowledged their existence.' [55] But at least the teacher seemed present. Kessel later watches the same coach teach a mixed group of children. With the girls, she writes, the coach has a resignation about him. 'He didn't seem to believe the girls were worth investing in.'

In addition body-image concerns often mean that girls (including me) don't want to participate in activity. This seeps into adulthood too. A survey by *Cosmopolitan* in 2015 found that the majority of women polled felt intimidated in the gym – and 14 per cent of those specifically dreaded men judging them.[56] It's not just the gym, either. The only part of running that I loathed when I started (and still do) is the sheer volume of men who see you as a target when you're out on the roads. Men have stopped me dead in my tracks, run alongside me, honked from cars and vans, driven slowly next to me; and, on one memorable occasion, grabbed me by the waist as I went past. I hate having to consider which roads to jog down, whether someone is drunk enough that they might lunge at you, or knowing that, because it's hot and you have to wear shorts, some big shot will feel like it's his God-given right to critique your outfit – as though he's judge on *Project Runway* and not, well, just a gross pervert.

Even as a prepubescent kid I worried about this kind of

intimidation. Rigid gender stereotypes had yet to be challenged back when I was at primary school, and boys would laugh if you so much as attempted to join in on the football pitch. Mildly discouraging, I found this kind of behaviour got much worse as a teenager feeling awkward about a newly developing body. In her brilliant book *Running Like a Girl*, about training for and then running a marathon, Alexandra Heminsley talks about having similar teenage antipathy towards exercise. 'My body, once a source of such fun, was now more of an unreliable straitjacket. When I wasn't fretting about how it looked I was worrying about what shape it might be next.'[57]

It's difficult to track accurately, but many experts believe that those put off by sport at school are much more likely to remain inactive as adults.[58] I went to the local gym aged sixteen, thinking that I should at least see if I'd been wrong to write off exercise entirely. On one visit, I was flirted with, berated for using a machine the wrong way, and laughed at in the weights room. I didn't set foot in a gym for fourteen years after that. An overreaction? Maybe, but I was already an insecure novice and the atmosphere I found was more than unpleasant, it was unwelcoming.

As you can see, I didn't take any steps that might have helped, and despite all my ridiculous mental safeguards, I was headed for what I assume a Victorian aunt would politely call 'a breakdown'.*

I left school, with no real idea of what to do next. Going to university away from home was out of the question, I was

---

* This is in no way a medical term, I just like it. It makes me feel like I've been locked away in a turret stuffed with cobwebs, wearing a wedding dress. Let me be.

too scared to leave. Scared of what was unclear, but I came up with my usual trusty excuses – London was too fun, campus life looked dull, I wanted to be different. Of all the things anxiety stopped me from doing, going to university away from home is the one I resent not doing the most. I spent my twenties holding onto my adolescence, slightly suspended in space. Perhaps university would've pushed me towards adulthood faster. Everyone I knew that went away flourished in a way that I did not – venturing into a new independent world; making new friends, choosing how to live for themselves.

Instead I stayed local, but even that wasn't safe enough for me. The university I picked was in the centre of the city. Even just enrolling was a terrifying day of holding down panic just long enough to get my student card. My dad had to meet me halfway through the morning just to give me a boost and to stop me fleeing in terror. I guess that means my dad came with me on my first day of university. As you can imagine, I'm feeling pretty cool right about now. Not as cool as I felt then though, obviously.

University went well, and I passed with a first easily. KIDDING. I dropped out after six months. I just couldn't do it. I couldn't face the panic I felt every time I had to go into town. I'd have huge panic attacks in lectures and have to leave. The weird thing about panic attacks is, although you feel like the whole room is looking at you, it's more likely that nobody has noticed a thing. But they would defeat me – the dangers seemed to be everywhere and I was exhausted from safeguarding against them. I'd be left dripping in sweat, exhausted and trembling, tearful that I was so useless.

My parents had by now figured out that something wasn't right and sent me to see a therapist who very calmly told me

I was having panic attacks and had generalised anxiety disorder (GAD, as in Oh my GAD I'm so anxious). It might seem absurd that it took me nineteen years to figure out that I had a mental-health problem, but it's more common than you might think. One in 4 people in the UK are estimated to experience mental illness in their lives, and it's not hard to imagine that many of them struggle alone, not getting a definite diagnosis or proper help. While writing this book, I spoke to a friend about mental illness and he disclosed that he'd recently been diagnosed with anxiety and depression (the two often go hand in hand). He's 34, and had lived for fifteen years thinking he just had a 'sad' mentality, and that there was nothing wrong with him. It took a crisis in his relationship to seek help, and he was genuinely surprised to find out he had an illness. Once it was confirmed, he began to get help. It was a relief to know that his life could be better, but I felt incredibly despondent that he'd just assumed that sadness was his lot. And his story is not rare.

Once I'd found out what was wrong with me, the panic attacks slacked off for a bit. It was as though knowing what was happening released some of the fear. Knowledge is power and all that. I knew I wouldn't die from one, so I didn't have them as much. If only it were that simple for all mental-health symptoms. But I was very embarrassed by the term 'anxiety' – having spent years trying to be the same as everyone else, it felt like a failure to have to acknowledge that I wasn't. Even if my difference wasn't my fault, or a weakness, it sure felt like it was. I made it a joke, always my first line of defence (and still my instinct to this day, you might have noticed), and tried to minimise it.

Though I now had some idea what I was dealing with, I

*still* failed to tackle in it any meaningful way. Perhaps I got confident – I knew what a panic attack was, and that felt like enough. I didn't spend much time looking into what other symptoms might accompany these attacks, or whether I might suffer with this disorder for the rest of my life. It felt like something I was merely trying on for size, wearing these worries until I properly grew up and grew out of them. I was given beta blockers, which were originally developed for heart problems but calm the physical side effects of panic – like a racing heart and sweaty palms. They are often taken by people who hate public speaking, and by musicians before a big performance. They're very effective on the body, but they didn't do anything for my racing mind. These tiny pills can't cure anxiety, or ease your fears; they just help a little bit with the day-to-day symptoms.

I dithered about for a bit, completely lost in the way that many nineteen-year-olds are. But then I made it to art school and had a fantastic year where I made friends and relaxed and thought that I'd shrugged off the fear for good. That sneaky anxiety had different ideas, of course. In my second year everything fell apart. It started small. I felt odd on the normal bus journey to college. Something quickly felt wrong, and the world began to look dark and menacing. I ended up walking into the building, walking out immediately and having the worst panic attack I'd ever had in the Uni car park. Only it felt worse than a normal panic attack. It wasn't merely that I was breathless or dizzy, something felt like it had flipped inside my brain and I had nothing to compare it to. My thoughts were whizzing along at a rate I'd never experienced. Words were sticking in my head, as though a record was stuck on repeat. Colours looked too bright – like strip lighting behind my eyes. Even my concerned friends looked different – like strangers wearing familiar masks. I sat in the car park, trying to shake off these strange new symptoms, gulping air and rubbing my hands together quickly and frantically.

Because I had no idea what my brain was doing, I went home almost immediately pleading a headache, and chalked it up to a blip. But I couldn't get on the bus the next day. Or the next. I missed college for a week and hid out at my family home, feeling wrong, with panic in my guts the moment I woke up. People often feel at their most anxious in the mornings, when their stress hormone – cortisol – surges. You wake up feeling as if you've already drunk three litres of coffee, and the doom feeling rushes in. It can make starting the day feel like the worst thing in the world, as though you just know whatever comes next will be too hard to cope with before you've even brushed your teeth.

And the weird feeling that my brain had flipped didn't cease. My thoughts were going haywire, dancing to a tune I couldn't hear and dancing badly – kicking parts of my skull, falling over and hurting my eyes. Anxiety sufferers will be well acquainted with 'what if' thoughts – when your brain posits questions to itself, often without any warning. These can be obvious ones like 'What if I faint in the meeting?' or 'What if nobody likes me?' and I was used to this kind of questioning. But the questions my brain was asking had turned so sinister. I had felt so odd that day in the car park, that I was very frightened that there was more to it than merely anxiety. So my brain asked the 'obvious' question – What if I'm going mad?

This is an intrusive thought. These are astoundingly common – we all have them. 'What if I push this old lady down the escalator?' would be one. These notions pop into our brains and surprise us with their weirdness, but they don't mean we want to push old ladies down escalators. In 1978, leading OCD expert and psychologist Stanley Rachman polled a group of healthy students and a group of his patients, and found that nearly everyone in both groups had experienced thoughts like this. Crucially though, those not affected by OCD could easily shrug off such questions without being disturbed or ascribing the thoughts any meaning or weight. The group of patients could not do this; instead, the thoughts would paralyse them, and they would ruminate and obsess about what the intrusive thought must mean. A person with anxiety, depression or OCD might think 'What if I push this old lady down the escalator?' and become convinced that they want to, worrying about whether that makes them a monster, or even a murderer. This can lead to a person inventing a complicated mental jigsaw to 'neutralise' such ideas. A person might have an intrusive thought and immediately have to conjure up an image of their family being safe, or think of a specific word to cancel it out.

My brain asked if I was mad, and naturally, I freaked out. A person without anxiety might laugh and ignore it. Not me! I stopped sleeping, and spent every possible minute tangling myself up in knots trying to reject this idea. The trouble is, the more you try and reassure yourself, the more your brain will one-up you. Sneaky brain, always able to terrify you more than you imagine.

Seemingly overnight, my 'what if' thoughts had gone from my usual 'What if the plane I'm on crashes?' worries to 'What if I think everyone's out to get me?' Both were fairly irrational, but one felt familiar and based on some grounding in reality.

The other felt impossible to prove or disprove – but my mind went into overdrive trying. I'd google symptoms, thoughts and statistics. I'd lie in bed turning the results over in my brain, overwhelmed with the barrage of ideas I was experiencing – it felt like thousands every second. 'What if I'm crazy?' 'What if I think everyone is out to get me?' 'What if I kill my sister?' 'What if the advice website I just clicked on is all wrong?' 'What if I'm dangerous?' 'Let me just go through all of those ideas again and argue with them.' Fucking exhausting.

These kinds of obsessive thoughts have been seen throughout human history – mainly in the form of religious scrupulosity. The importance of faith and the fear of the Church seen in previous eras make this understandable. Intrusive thoughts about God would strike terror into those afflicted. In 1691, Bishop John Moore published a pamphlet about these thoughts, which made me smile when I first read it. Not only did he describe my millennial brain with uncanny accuracy, but the route he suggested to tackle these thoughts is one I have heard from countless living experts and modern books on the subject:

'When you find these thoughts creeping upon you, be not mightily dejected . . . Neither violently struggle with them; since experience doth teach that they increase and swell by vehement opposition; but dissipate and waste away, & come to nothing when they are neglected, and we do not much concern ourselves about them . . . It is not therefore a furious combat with melancholy thoughts, which will but weaken and sink the body, and to make the case worse, but a gentle application of such comfortable things as restore the strength, and recruit the languishing spirit that must quash and disperse these disorderly tumults in the head.'[59]

Who would have thought a bishop alive during the Great Fire of London would bring me such relief?

I've never fully expanded on this period of my life to anyone. Mainly because, as I have said before, I was ashamed and embarrassed. I've touched on some of the thoughts to my nearest and dearest. I remember one night hysterically sobbing on the bed as my dad tried to calm me down. 'But maybe I think everyone is a robot,' I wept, as he reassured me that I didn't. But I wasn't sure he was right and I could see that his daughter blurting out such odd ideas was probably too much for a non-professional to cope with. So I didn't really go into detail with people. Instead I'd just say I was going mad, and let people take from that what they wanted.

But you're paying for this book (I hope – don't nick it or anything). And maybe you're thinking that my privileged-woman anxiety isn't all that crippling. So I'll try and be brutally honest about my thought process at this fucking awful moment in my life.

In the space of about three days after the car park moment, this is where my brain went:

*That was scary and new, maybe it's not anxiety.*

*If it's not anxiety, am I going mad?*

*What is madness? I think it's psychosis.*

*Oh fuck, I'm psychotic.*

*Psychotic people think that the TV is sending them messages. Do I think that?*

*No, of course not. But then I've just watched TV and wondered if I do. So I MUST THINK IT.*

*No, you don't because you know you have anxiety and this is just fear.*

*No, I feel detached and strange and everyone in the world looks fake and unreal.*

*Do I think I'm in* The Truman Show? *Do I think everyone is acting around me?*

*No, that's just derealisation, you've had it before.*

*But I keep thinking it. I DO think that – so I'm mad. I'll have to go and live in an asylum and I'll begin hearing voices.*

*Am I hearing voices? Is that voice in my head as I fall asleep a sign of my descent?*

*I'm trying to catch my friends out, trying to prove they're acting, even though I know rationally that they're not. Do I really not trust anybody?*

*Does the world look like a fake movie set? It's all flat and strange. What if I think it's all faked and nothing is real?*

*What if I kill my parents because I think they're robots and I don't know I've done it?*

*What if I live in a simulation? What if I'm actually dead? Let me just go through all of those ideas again and argue with them for hours.*

There were thousands more of these thoughts, and I'm not exaggerating when I say I didn't think of anything else in my waking hours. Not a single other thing. I couldn't eat. I couldn't sleep – instead I would close my eyes and see surreal cartoon characters fornicating behind my eyelids (hypnagogic hallucinations). There was no sleeping when they were shocking me with acts of depravity that would make a porn star blush.

The frequency and intensity of the thoughts made me feel as though waves were repeatedly crashing over me, giving me no time to recover before the next assault. I had no time to recover from one scary 'what if' question before another would hit. I didn't take the good bishop's advice, and instead spent all my time trying to argue with the thoughts, or refute them, accept them, shake them off. But nothing worked. My head was a tangled mess of irrational information and I would subsequently hyperventilate, weep, and retch every time a new thought entered my brain, as though I could expel them from my very being.

And my general anxiety wasn't going anywhere either. The exhaustion of fighting my own thoughts didn't stop my whole body from humming with adrenaline. I couldn't eat anything, and my stomach churned – I felt so weak I could barely muster the strength to do anything. Not that I had anything to do. I couldn't go back to college, I didn't want to see anyone. I just lay in bed, occasionally getting up and crying as I wandered around the house aimlessly, deep in my brain, thinking, thinking, thinking.

At this point, I was completely unable to help myself. My sister kindly refers to this period as 'the time you stared at walls'. So others had to step in. I am privileged to have a family who were able to throw money at the problem. My GP, who had previously prescribed me beta blockers, offered me a very old-fashioned antidepressant drug with sedative qualities, and warned that if I wanted therapy it would mean six months on a waiting list. I cried with the hopelessness of that information. Almost every day I think of the people up and down the country who are suicidal, desperate, lost; and who can't get access to the services that might help them in time.

Mental-health provision has always been stretched in the UK, but recent cuts have not helped the many people with serious problems who are not being seen soon enough, or by the right department, despite the government pledging an extra £1bn for mental-health treatment.[60][61][62] The NHS introduced the Improving Access to Psychological Therapies (IAPT) programme in 2008, which announced in 2016 the aim of getting 75 per cent of people with mental-health problems seen within six weeks and 95 per cent within a maximum time frame of eighteen weeks.[63] While this goal is better than nothing, try explaining to a frantic and frightened person that they have to stay as they are for a possible four months. A friend of mine has been in and out of hospital for mental-health issues, and her story is one of cancelled sessions; waiting lists; travelling for miles to a hospital nowhere near her home and being wrongly diagnosed because she never sees the same doctor. That's not to say the NHS isn't trying its best, it is – it just doesn't have the resources to actually treat everyone properly.

I was lucky enough to go and see an incredibly kind psychiatrist almost immediately, who listened as I told him every single terrible thought I had endured, argued with him that I must be mad, and cried inconsolably. He explained that what I was dealing with was still anxiety, and that the obsessive thoughts that I was having were still a part of that (I told you OCD wasn't about extreme tidiness). He gave me anti-depressants, which I'd been vehemently opposed to (they felt like a defeat), but which I took because I wanted to die and somehow still knew that this wasn't normal. Bryony Gordon describes this reluctance well in her memoir *Mad Girl*, saying that reading the leaflet regarding possible side effects was daunting ('as long as *War and Peace*'), but she didn't care because she'd rather have had osteoarthritis than OCD at that moment. I remember thinking the same. That sort of puts paid to the idea that those of us who take antidepressants are searching for some imaginary effortless high.

'"Hope" is the thing with feathers –' according to Emily Dickinson, 'That perches in the soul.' In the weeks that followed, I crawled very slowly towards some kind of weak light. As the drugs began to work, I was packed off to see friends at university in Nottingham. I sat on the train numbly gazing out of the window, as the intrusive thoughts shuffled through my head. 'What if I think the scenery is fake?' 'What if my friends try to poison me?' 'Why would they do that? This is mad.' 'You're not mad, this is anxiety . . .'

I managed the visit. I managed a few visits to the shops. I even spent a night at the pub. But I was battered by this break in my brain. I felt that my mind had been irredeemably damaged by the thoughts, by the anxiety, by the thoughts of death. Even though the thoughts were receding slowly, I had no idea how to carry on with life as if nothing had happened. I was still seeking reassurance, still googling symptoms madly, still frightened.

I was furious too. Furious that I'd been saddled with this fear which, on good days, sat in my stomach, and on bad days seeped through my entire being, as though my body was merely a host for a terrifying gremlin who hated me. Everyone else around me made it look like life could be fun and care-free. Why couldn't I, even just for a day?

Yet even as my brain got quieter, I grew depressed. Sadness was thrown over my anxiety like a wet blanket over a fire. Everything felt hopeless, and I had huge feelings of guilt about being so worthless. Even my dog made me cry. I'd look into his rheumy eyes and think he deserved a better owner.

I'd been pulled through a crisis by those who loved me, because I couldn't get through it alone. But I hadn't been able to help myself at all. I was tentatively on the other side, but there was no relief to be found there either. I was twenty, with no further education or job. I was more fearful than ever. I wondered if I'd ever truly break free from my worried mind, but it didn't seem likely. Life seemed to have stopped before I'd had a chance to really give it a proper go.

4K — IS IT TOO
LATE TO TRY?

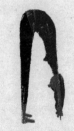

I'm running with my sister for the first time. It's the first time I've run with anyone. My sister is tall and freakishly strong, and she's always mocked me for my small stature (I'm five foot seven, only short by my giant family's terms) and my inability to arm-wrestle her or open jars with ease. She picked up running with ease a few years before me, running half marathons with gusto after drinking a bottle of red wine the night before. She goes swimming in lakes in January while I stand on the banks in two coats laughing at her. We are very different in how we approach exercise. But here we are, one summer's day, pacing each other (near enough), and I'm even managing to talk as I struggle along. We've ducked out as the rest of the family sleep off a big lunch, and we weave through the village where my parents live, passing chickens and sheep grazing in fields, jogging past the local pub where we used to eat as children. We hit country roads, and end up running next to hedgerows as we pick up mud with our feet. I feel secretly bursting to be able to keep up with my long-legged sibling. While I've always found her jokes about my anxious, frail nature very funny, it still feels incredible to be able to do something with her that takes power and stamina. As we go, we talk about the past few months, and I absorb the praise she gives me for trying to tackle my anxiety. Then, ever the younger (and more competitive) sister, she decides I'm going too slowly and picks up her own pace. After a few loops back to me, we head back home, and I discover I managed to run for twenty-four minutes without checking my progress once. I'd previously thought that running was a solely solitary pursuit, something to do sheepishly and almost apologetically. But that first run with my sister flew by, and I resolved not to hide my growing passion from other runners, despite my slow gait and inability to arm-wrestle.

Why do I have anxiety? What causes it? It can be hard to have an illness that is so often misunderstood, but it's also hard when so little about anxiety can easily be explained – even by experts. The NHS gives several reasons why a person might have an anxiety issue like GAD, including:

- An overactivity in areas of the brain involved in emotions and behaviour
- An imbalance of the brain chemicals serotonin and noradren-aline, which are involved the regulation of mood
- The genes you inherit – it's estimated that you're five times more likely to develop GAD if you have a close relative with the disorder.
- A history of stressful or traumatic experiences [64]

There are loads more of course. Biological factors, social factors and psychological factors all have many strands and layers which can contribute. Modern life is full of stresses which can easily make mental-health conditions worse. Long working hours, commuting, finances, loneliness and inequality – they can all make a person who's prone to anxious thoughts or low mood rapidly deteriorate. We live less communally, our family units atomised. Our circle of friends and loved ones is often scattered – in 2017, there were 3.9 million people living alone between the ages of 16 and 64. That's a lot of people at risk of isolation.

Poverty is also a huge factor in people's quality of mental health. The Centre for Social Justice (CSJ), a conservative think tank, found that children and adults from the lowest bracket (the fifth quintile) of household income groups are three times more likely to have common mental-health problems than those in the richest bracket (the first quintile).[65] They are nine times as likely to have psychotic disorders. Their report identifies six factors which make low income groups vulnerable to mental illness:

- Unemployment
- The lack of opportunities
- The likelihood of getting into debt
- A lack of qualifications
- Family breakdown
- Addiction issues

In addition to those living in low-income families, black and minority ethnic groups (BAME) in the UK suffer disproportionately from mental illness. People in these groups are more likely to be diagnosed and admitted to hospital, more likely to experience a poor outcome from treatment and more likely to disengage from mainstream mental-health services. This isn't surprising when you learn that people from BAME groups are more likely to be sectioned (detained under mental-health legislation, sometimes against a person's will) than their white counterparts. Alongside this, 'black people are 40 per cent more likely to be turned away than white people when they ask for help from mental health services,' according to the CSJ.[66]

So there are reasons why some people are hit harder than others with mental-health problems. And some of the gaps which people are liable to slip through could be fixed, with the right funding, resources, education and cultural under-standing. There are many things in our society that we need to put right, and many people we are failing. And sometimes, addressing a specific factor can go some way to helping recovery. But when you're suffering, sometimes valid reasons don't mean a thing.

Right down at the bottom of the NHS list above comes one last reason for anxiety – and it's the one I always end up thinking about: 'Many people will develop GAD for no apparent reason.'[67] The same thing can be said about OCD (is it caused by trauma? physical illness? genetics?), social anxiety, and a host of other mental illnesses. And that can be frustrating to live with. We will some of us never know why we have anxiety or depression, and if we don't know the origin of the problem, then how can we hope to 'fix' it? This uncer-tainty made me tie myself up in knots for a while when I was struggling. My grandfather was an anxious man, very concerned with health issues (both real and imagined). Was that all it took for me to be so unhappy? And if so, why wasn't my dad, or my sister? Was it because I had tonsillitis when I was younger? Even my mum got in on it – was it because she left me with a babysitter at two months old? It made her feel guilty. It still does. Recent research has found brain cells in mice that appear to control anxiety – does my hippocampus hold the key?

It felt important to isolate the original cause of my problems, important enough to go over my early childhood with a keen therapist who seemed to think we'd find the answer if I just worked hard enough at it. I wanted to, but it didn't happen. It was enough to make me research the possible link between physical illness and the onset of mental-health problems. I researched brain chemicals and fell down holes on the internet that suggested ridiculous reasons – made by desperate people like me, wishing for something they could ascribe it to and therefore address. Cut out dairy! If only it could be that easy.

Despite it sometimes feeling like anxiety is a thoroughly modern illness, it has been around as long as we have, though it's been called many different things. It was recognised in a religious sense long ago – in the context of sin, redemption and the judgement of God. Hippocrates mentioned phobias in his texts – specifically of flutes. Existentialist philosophers like Heidegger believed anxiety was caused by the realisation that our existence is finite. Which is cheery.

Is it comforting to know that people experienced similar suffering hundreds of years ago? I guess that depends on the person. I always took some solace that the great thinkers of years gone by also struggled with intrusive thoughts and physical panic. But it also shows how little progress we've made in ridding ourselves of anxiety. And that's less heartening. Especially since so many of us suffer from it now.

Life can never be an uninterrupted journey of unwavering happiness, where problems are handled with stoicism and a smile. It never was, despite what some tabloids would have you believe about the war years. There will always be sadness and worry mixed in with the good.

But anxiety is on the rise – at least, that's what the media would have us believe. I'm always cynical when I see headlines frequently refer to the 'anxiety epidemic', as though mental illness was contagious and likely to turn us into neurotic zombies. But despite my annoyance at much mental-health coverage, statistics do seem to indicate a global uptick. Figures from the World Health Organisation for 2016 show that the incidence of common mental disorders has increased around the world. Between 1990 and 2013, the number of people suffering from anxiety and/or depression went up by nearly 50 per cent, from 416 million to 615 million.[68]

So it's understandable that you might feel as though anxiety is more prevalent in the modern age. Alongside an actual rise in the disorder, these figures are probably boosted by a mix of things – a better definition of what anxiety and depression actually mean, quicker diagnosis, and official figures being available – all of which are good things when you think about it.

But even if there is clearer data available on mental illness, even if you know that biological factors were stacked against you from the beginning, or can see that a traumatic event kicked it all off, does it help? Part of living with mental illness is confronting this seeming injustice, and accepting that your number came up when they were doling out anxiety. Knowing that mental illness has been a part of life through the ages might mean very little, but knowing you're not alone is something else. I might never have an answer as to why I was given the capacity for great worry, but being increasingly open about it has meant meeting others who understand, and who come with empathy and goodwill. Not being alone with your scary and sad thoughts is one of the best ways to hold such thoughts at bay. For some people, that might mean opening up to friends and family. For others, it could mean finding a support group – in your community or online. Don't just sit and ask, 'Why me?' as I have done so many times. Go and talk to others. 'Us' is far better than 'me' when it comes to mental health.

I don't want to bore you into submission, dear and valued reader, by documenting the rest of my twenties. There's a good reason we all (well, most of us) nod at the old cliché that your thirties are the reward for your earlier years. Most people find their twenties difficult – and if you don't, what were you doing? Were you already forging a great career and getting early nights? I hate you – and I was no different. Oprah Winfrey once said of this period: 'When I was in my twenties, I was a lost soul. Your twenties are about finding your soul.'[69]

I don't know about lost soul, but my anxiety definitely didn't go away. Nay, it got worse. I took the antidepressants, I went to see a few therapists, with differing results. One insisted I talk about my childhood incessantly to unlock the problem. Another doodled a lot while I talked, which I found both hilarious and intimidating – was I so boring? (Probably.) In one memorable and excruciating instance, I went to see an eerily handsome man who wore loafers and a pinky ring and made me lie down on an enormous leather recliner and talk to my five-year-old self. 'Soothe her, Isabella, hold her hand and tell her not to be afraid.' I'm not exaggerating when I say I started getting physical panic signs from the horror I felt at this absurdity. After giving him a cheque for a LUDICROUS amount of money, I fled from his office and never went back. My five-year-old self can go whistle.

I worked as a journalist, but felt lacking, stupid and insecure a lot of the time. I never put myself forward for promotion or raised my voice much. This might not be just because of my anxiety, by the way – a recent study by several leading universities asked 985,000 people in forty-eight countries to rate the statement: 'I see myself as someone who has high self-esteem.' The researchers found that across the board, men have higher self-esteem than women. Beyond that, I couldn't leave home for years, and even then I moved across the road, much to the mirth of friends. It's funny, except it's not really. I couldn't spread my wings and create an independent life; my brain wouldn't let me. What if, what if, what if? whirred my mind. Stay close to home. Don't risk it. What was 'it' exactly? Everything.

I guess I lived a sort of half-life. I was able to work, which makes me incredibly lucky, since 300,000 people with long-term mental-health issues lose their jobs each year, according to a study commissioned by the Prime Minister published in October 2017. My boss was kind about my sudden moments of anxiety, and she made sure to try and understand, even if I didn't. I socialised within my own limits. I didn't stray far – hard to, really, when I wouldn't even take the Tube. I stayed within the confines I set for myself, and painted on that small canvas. I kidded myself that that was enough – sometimes when you say something enough you start to believe it. My anxiety ebbed and flowed. Sometimes I grew cocky and would think I was over the big crash of my late teens, and inevitably I would then be crushed by another low period. I had a very doomed love affair which ran until I was about twenty-six, and the end of that relationship sent me straight back to all the same symptoms and horror that I'd had six years previously.

Once again, I was consumed by a cycle of panic, intrusive thoughts and near-hysteria at every waking moment. It was ferocious, and much worse than before. Once again, I went back to the gentle psychiatrist I'd seen before and insisted he commit me. As before, he was kind and patient. 'Take it from this old man, Isabella,' he said. 'Lost affairs of the heart produce the worst pain you can feel.'

Ooof, I cried.

So I took more drugs, I stared at walls, I retreated. I remember my mum dragging me to the shops to cheer me up, and I cried as I looked at shoes (maybe that should be the title of my memoir). I remember my dad soothing me to sleep as if I were a helpless child, which I was. Except I wasn't really. It was all wrong, upside down, a dark version of youth. The crash which I had so dreaded happening again, had roared back to remind me that I would likely never be free of fear. And for all the support, all the kindness and love I was so fortunate to receive, I secretly knew that this meant I couldn't really recover this time. Not properly. The anxiety I'd stored up about feeling that level of panic again felt completely justified. I'd been an ostrich with my head in the sand, hoping I'd be OK if I just stayed small, didn't push myself, never experienced risk. But I'd risked, because you can't avoid it, and I'd fallen. I begged to be committed, to be sectioned, anything to quit this life which I found too hard. I felt like I hadn't been given the requisite armour for the game, and I didn't want to play.

If you're getting a little annoyed with my obtuse and stupid refusal to tackle my problems, that's OK. With the benefit of hindsight, I'm still angry with myself. I made things so much harder than they had to be. I did everything you're not supposed to do when diagnosed with a mental illness – hid it, tried to argue with it, let it take over. But so many people do. It's not really a big surprise though, is it? Not when you consider how mental illness has been covered in the press for years, and when you think about how people casually talk about 'psychos' and 'mad people'. Then there's the classic assumption that you'll inevitably face from a few people in your life, who view depression or anxiety as a weakness, and who make it clear that you probably could just pull yourself together. And while these views are fading somewhat, they aren't gone completely, and I don't blame anyone who feels as though it's too risky to open up about their problems. But ultimately, talking is the only way we'll stamp out prejudice entirely. And equally importantly, the more we talk about mental-health problems, the more people will know how to get effective help, and fewer people will rely on their own stupid coping mechanisms. Writing this book has cheered me, since so many young people have told me that they sought help early. It's brilliant to hear that new generations aren't waiting and hiding, and I'm filled with admiration for those who look for help immediately. But there's still so much to be done, and bravely seeking help is no use if the resources aren't there to give it to you as soon as you ask for it.

Back in my cycle of ignoring my anxiety, minimising it to others and hoping it would go away, I met a man. He didn't seem too keen on me initially, which of course made it all the more interesting. I quietly hung around, seeing him when he suggested it, staying back when he signalled a lack of enthusiasm. I never demanded he take me seriously, given my lack of self-worth and my utter gratitude that someone would like me even a little bit. Proper embarrassing doormat behaviour, and I'm cringing slightly as I type. I just felt strongly that this grown-up man, several years older than me, would complete my life in a way that I hadn't been able to. Nothing else had pushed me into real life as I saw it – maybe a partner could? A completely ridiculous notion – how can you have a proper relationship if you're not a proper person? Nevertheless, I persevered.

I once watched a very trashy rom-com in which a character urges her best friend to make a change in her life. One line stuck with me, and apologies for the paraphrasing but I'm not going to watch it again (OK, I might). 'Some people reach a crossroads in their life – and either they choose to power on and do something scary, or they become shell people. When you meet those people, you wonder – what happened to them to make them like that?'

It stuck with me because I knew I was a shell person. Nice outer demeanour, could do a good impression of being a fully formed adult, occasionally funny, but that was all there was to me. Look inside and there wasn't anything else, no hidden mass. Just a shell. A nice shell, but that's not enough. Friends at that time might read all of this with surprise or even mild disbelief. 'She wasn't that bad,' I guess some might say. 'She wasn't sad.' But that's what you get good at when you've lived with anxiety for years. You hide it, gloss over it, dismiss with convoluted excuses any activity which might frighten you. If you've ever had a panic attack, you'll know that it seems like everyone in the world can see it happening – as though you're a bright red, honking fire truck in a quiet library. But in reality, you're like a duck, serene on the water. The furious activity all takes place under water, as you paddle and kick.

You can do a good job of looking like more than a shell. And I persisted with this romance. He was a smart, solid, kind guy, with none of the problems I had (this was another mad thought – everyone has problems, everyone has weird issues, of course he did). And his interest eventually grew. To the point where he proposed after three months of proper solid dating. And I was thrown into complete panic. This is what I wanted, surely – a normal relationship to provide me with all the strength and character that I lacked. If I couldn't be a fully rounded individual, then someone else could tack onto me and bump up my average. But it was all so rushed, so decisive, that my reaction to his proposal was muted at best. I said yes, then got on the bus and went home. Where I promptly burst into tears and sought reassurance from my mum (she said it was normal – cheers, Mum). But then how could it feel right? Nothing else did.

One of the biggest problems with anxiety is that it makes you unsure as to what is merely irrational worry, and what is legitimate. Once you know you have severe anxiety, you get used to the fact that most of your shit can be chalked up to the illness. Instead of assuming I'm having a stroke, I usually realise, 'Oh, this is panic again.' When I feel faint; when I feel hungry; when I feel cold; when I feel sleepy; when I feel stomach pains or when I feel teary; I tend to trust Occam's Razor – that the simplest explanation is usually the better one. It's a strange thing, no longer trusting your instinct that something might be wrong. You never know if anxiety is masking something serious, or whether the symptoms are cooked up by it. It's a slippery thing, mimicking other illnesses if you're worried about them, and throwing up problems that could be anything. Currently I have back pain. My mind is having a lot of fun conjuring up crazy theories about it. It's *back pain*. Basically the whole world has it. But my brain is directing me towards several other suggestions, all of which are more exotic. As you might imagine, doctors love me – there's a lot of 'while I'm here . . .' at my appointments.

The internet – don't google health problems, folks, it only makes you think you have a tropical disease – is full of people who have anxiety diagnoses from professionals, but who still worry about symptoms which might indicate cancer, diabetes, psychosis, or a myriad of other things. In the back of their minds, they usually know it's their anxiety, but they can't quite be sure. All of this is to say, yeah, it's probably that, but the worry doesn't stop. You have to strike up a balance between not ignoring feelings and instincts, and not being led by them. I haven't fully mastered this.

So I felt anxious as hell about getting married and I didn't know if that was because that's how I always felt or because my brain was trying to be a pal for once, and warn me off the idea. I spent a lot of time trying to figure it out, but how could I? I'd never tried to understand how my anxiety worked – not really; and I didn't trust my own mind one way or another. Sometimes I was adamant that it was all fine, and my worries were irrational; and other times I was quietly certain that my relationship wasn't right. I didn't really mention this to anyone – the wheels were in motion, everyone liked my boyfriend; I was around what I thought was 'the right age'; and I couldn't think of a reason to blow up my life and the security the relationship promised. Besides, I reasoned that, either way, the fault lay at my door.

So we got married. I had time to get used to the idea, and I was genuinely committed to it. There were some red flags beforehand but my self-esteem was pants, so I put up with a few things I would never dream of allowing now. The wedding was GREAT, by the way. I highly recommend doing it if you have a nice partner and want to wear something fun. We had a big, boozy, relaxed day which included my dogs for part of it, and involved a ton of tiramisu. I don't know much about how to make a marriage work (read: nothing), but the day itself can be really fun! Friends, family, music, and everyone has to say how great you look. Have a think about it. And do invite me, I still love them, despite mine being a huge harbinger of doom. For the love of God though, have it in the late afternoon. Nobody wants to start drinking champagne at 11 a.m. At least, not if you still want to be awake at 11 p.m.

I wasn't anxious at all on the day, as it turned out. I'm anxious on boring Sundays, but apparently not on the day I get married and have had consuming conflicting opinions about the whole thing. My brain is a huge troll. As we headed off on honeymoon, I sort of thought maybe the wedding was the remedy, and that I'd be OK from here on out. NOPE! I spent my first night sleepless, feeling spacey and strung out and strange. People looked odd, I swore the floor was moving, the colours were off. And it didn't get any better. In the run-up to the wedding I'd nursed a huge fear of developing anaphylactic shock – from food, from make-up, from hair dye. It consumed me in the way the mad thoughts did (irrational thoughts seem to have a tendency to jump about and latch on to new fears, which can take you by surprise and freak you out – never a dull moment), and I spent a lot of time breathing in and out oddly: to check that I could. I was stung by a bee and had to sleep for three hours after a huge panic attack. My honeymoon was dogged by this stupid and pathetic fear – though I never said it out loud, as usual. On top of this, I felt like I might faint at any moment and disassociation crept back in. My new husband looked like a stranger, and I felt like an automaton. Sounds like the beginning of an amazing love story, huh?

On one of the last days, in a busy shopping street, I begged my husband not to go and get a coffee without me. Not because I was so wrapped up in marital bliss that I couldn't bear to lose him, but because I was too scared to be on my own in public. Aged 29, just married, with a dog and a husband and presumably a pension somewhere, I couldn't be on my own for two minutes. That's where a lifetime of anxiety and ignoring that anxiety had led me to. I felt so pathetic and I'm sure he thought I was too.

Some people thrive on other people needing them – their vulnerability makes the other person feel stronger. But that's not what an anxious person needs. It's not what anyone needs really. As much as you might want someone to support you and shield you, it only makes your brain more fearful. It enables your mind to whisper, 'See – even your loved ones think life is scary and dangerous for you. Best just sit here and not risk going out.'

But anxiety makes other people react differently. Some people tell you to buck up; some look at you like you might break; some tell you they worry all the time too and you just nod your head and smile at their attempts to relate. (Did *you* ever cry worrying that you'd killed your sister because you walked on the wrong slice of pavement and incurred the wrath of some evil spirit? Obviously, my sister was fine and my mind was just being an arsehole. But do go on about how you also feel jittery on planes.)

One guy got an actual erection when I told him I was having a panic attack. Imagine. Being aroused by someone else's fears. He tried to put my hand on it as if I'd be grateful. I still can't imagine a shittier reaction to anxiety but do let me know if you've had one!

Anyway, I'm getting sidelined. Avoid *that* guy. And don't let people encourage your anxiety out of misguided love or a need to feel better about themselves. And many people will do this, it sucks. Learn the signs and get out early.

Of course, you're only getting my side here. But here it is. I loved him. I thought it was going OK. I was certainly resolved that we'd stick it out and work at it whatever happened. But I was a secret shell-person and getting very bad at hiding it. It's difficult to agree to long-term plans when you're scared of going to the supermarket at the top of the road. I keep referencing this supermarket, but only because it's such a strong marker of how stuck I was. It's not because they're paying me.

We muddled on until Christmas, and then we started unravelling. Or maybe we already were but events applied more pressure. My husband was in a scary car accident which shook us both, and traumatised him. Though he was physically unhurt, he retreated into himself, his mood dimming and his usual good nature disappearing.

He was adamant that he was fine, and despite all evidence to the contrary, I didn't push it. I thought it would pass, that he was experiencing a moment of sadness, but I was horribly mistaken. A weekend away culminated in me crying in a fancy restaurant with real silver plates, asking him to be nicer to me. I began asking that a lot. I'd selfishly assumed I was the broken element in the partnership, and it was naive in the extreme to imagine I would always get to be the one being looked after. He needed help but, like so many people who find themselves depressed or anxious, he wouldn't ask for it or discuss it. Like I say, nobody is 'solid', nobody is totally sorted, and I stupidly looked for someone who seemed to be more in control than me. Turns out, I found someone who also had vulnerabilities and worries. And I couldn't help at all.

So now we were both miserable. He hadn't realised how scared I was, and I hadn't realised that he might have fallen into some darkness of his own. And he wouldn't talk about it, or couldn't, and I didn't want to explode the mine just sitting in our bedroom, so we went on with this guesstimation of a marriage, while I got more and more anxious and he got more and more angry and we slept facing away from each other.

By now, I was experiencing agoraphobia on a fairly severe level. I was frequently batting away intrusive thoughts and I was having panic attacks again. I couldn't take public transport, or go into town, or try out new experiences. I had to take two weeks off work because my brain got stuck in the old familiar loop and all the distress flooded back. I couldn't see how this had re-emerged again, and I was furious. I didn't see the trigger, which became glaringly clear soon afterwards. My marriage was failing.

I read an interview with the former Arsenal football player Tony Adams recently, where he said that his marriage works because his wife and he don't actually need each other. They love each other, but they would also be perfectly fine on their own. Their choice to be together is a deliberate one, not based on needing support or money or reassurance from somebody else. He no longer needs to be propped up by another person, and I understand this approach now. I had muddied the waters between love and need. I had looked for reassurance and instead I got increasingly short shrift, lessening affection and coldness. And I probably deserved a lot of it.

The day my husband left was the first day I had gone to see a new therapist, at his insistence. I came back hopeful, with cupcakes and balloons for my husband's birthday. I was going to tell him that I felt things could get better; that the nice therapist had assured me that, with work, I could slough off my anxieties and be a better wife, a better adult. But he sat at the table, with cupcakes uneaten, and told me that he was leaving me. I've described how it felt to hear that already; how I begged and pleaded and cried. But none of that worked; it turned out he'd been planning to leave for a long time, and had found a place to go weeks before. His choice was made, and I had no option but to catch up. 'We should never have got married,' were the last words I remember him saying to me. I also remember a real moment of gasping for breath, as though in a bad movie. The dog actually cried. And then my husband was gone.

The humiliation was total. We'd failed, but mainly I'd failed. I'd failed to be someone that could do what other people seem to do every day around the world – love and be loved. Because of many things, because relationships are complicated and human beings messy; but mainly I just blamed my anxiety. I felt tainted by it.

Almost everyone on earth has had a shitty break-up, and I am not special in dealing with anxiety alongside it. I handled the initial pain like most people do, even though I don't remember very much about the first couple of weeks. There were no inspirational quotes that gave me strength, no empowering music that made me feel like it would be OK. I just remember lying on the floor a lot (maybe just to ensure that it wouldn't treacherously shift even further).

The funny thing was, in the days that followed, I no longer felt as anxious. I felt a host of other shitty things, including anger and sadness; but not predominantly anxiety. There was a perverse relief in tanking everything so badly – I almost felt fearless – with nothing left to care about, I didn't have to be afraid I'd lose it. It turned out the marriage had made it all worse, not better. I suddenly felt restless – I wanted to do *something*. And because I'm not Bear Grylls or Amelia Earhart, I didn't go on an incredible brave global adventure, I just went for a run.

That first run I took up and down the alley was fuelled mainly by anger. I wanted to dramatically break out of my head, and I didn't know how to. Short of screaming and punching something, I thought moving as fast as I could might work. Turns out, I couldn't move very fast but it still felt like *something*. When I'd finished my three minutes huffing and puffing, I limped home feeling I'd sort of achieved my aim. I felt physically awful, but I'd pushed aside my thoughts for a moment. I'd gotten out of the misery cycle I'd been in since well before my husband left, and done something different – something nobody else knew about but me.

Sometimes, when you're at the end of your tether, it can only take one thing to make a difference. When you're so low, even a small change can provide a glimpse of hope. When I cast around and asked people for the things they tried when going through hard times, I got a range of answers: some funny, some obvious and some plain eccentric. Box sets were a favourite – binge-watching *The West Wing* on repeat (I can also recommend this); as was reading – books, magazines, the newspapers. Communal exercises were vouched for – learning an instrument in a group of beginners was mentioned, as was an old-fashioned knitting circle. An ex-colleague volunteered for as many charities and organisations as possible until all his time was taken up looking after others and he had no time to dwell on his own problems. Cooking also seemed popular: one respondent told me she ate potato gratin every day until she felt better, another cooked every chicken recipe he could think up. A photo sent by a stranger on social media alerted me to their amazing Lego habit, formed after a break-down. Pottery was another one, sculpting something, making something. Creating, not destroying.

People also told me about bigger challenges – trips to the Himalayas, silent meditation retreats and signing up for ultimate marathons. Those challenges have my admiration, but also would've seemed unattainable to me. But mainly people said exercise. Long walks – taken with no end goal or route – as one friend described it so well: 'Walking! Walking aimlessly for hours and hours, listening to music, stopping to people-watch. Sitting on benches, if it's sunny, closing your eyes and letting the sun warm your face.' Yoga to focus the mind and relax the body, boxing to get rid of adrenaline and anger. And running. Running came up a lot, so I wasn't very original in my choice – but I was obviously onto something.

Life didn't change, I kept on going to work; kept on crying

in the toilets; kept on running away from the looks on people's faces when I had to explain that my marriage was already over. I would call my husband and ask him if he'd changed his mind (spoiler alert: no, never). I packed all his stuff up as the dog watched warily, whining as I manically stuffed shirts into bin bags and books into old cardboard boxes. He came to pick them up and I noticed his wedding ring was gone. It turned out that he'd been looking for the exit long before I'd noticed. It amazes me what we refuse to see. My lovely sister came and stayed a lot – without me noticing, she sort of moved in and kept me getting up in the morning, made me shower, made me eat. I couldn't bypass the break-up, or ignore all my long-cultivated anxieties, but I could break out of it for a few minutes a day when I pulled on my old trainers, snuck out of the house after dark and headed to the alleyway where I had run that first day.

I kept heading back to the same starting place. I kept running to the same song. I felt out of breath and elephantine at every attempt. But I noticed that I was running for longer, that I would stop less and that I would even let the ridiculously angry song I relied on to lead into another track.

And I noticed physical changes too. I was sleeping better, not just staring at the ceiling while my sister slept next to me, and I drew some small comfort from her regular breathing and warmth. A simple reassurance that not everything had been ripped away from me. I wasn't hit with a huge adrenaline rush whenever I had an intrusive thought or moment of panic. I wasn't crying the moment I woke up. Progress! Well, of sorts.

I wasn't thinking clearly about very much at this point. Every day felt pretty gruelling, and it was as much as I could do to get up and go to work. I certainly wasn't seriously trying to alleviate my worries long term, or find a cure-all, but even I could see that my nightly jogs were lessening the load I felt in the immediate aftermath of my marriage collapse.

On the fourth night of running (I feel like a fraud saying running sometimes, given that I was mainly shuffling at this stage), I reached the end of the alleyway and didn't stop. It might not seem like a big step to some, but I was so scared of going out alone and stepping out of my 'safe' zone, that I felt like I was going to New Zealand. I emerged out onto a main road and cautiously continued, convinced that every passer-by and every driver would be laughing at my slow gait. This is a common fear for beginners – you are certain that you are being trailed by a beacon which screams 'I am new to this and doing it badly, please mock me.' The only advice I can give you is that you really aren't. I didn't run for the first thirty years of my life. I never noticed any of you – the beginners, the amazing sprinters – not one of you. And if I did, it was only to marvel that you wanted to, you know, actually get up off the sofa and move fast. You have to shrug it off and believe me here: most people don't look up from their phones anyway (which is a new problem when you start running, believe me; more on this later.)

Nobody batted an eyelid. Nobody screamed in abject horror. And I didn't fall down in a dead faint from fear. I ran an extra five minutes that night and went home elated, feeling like I'd tackled a hurdle I'd been eyeing up for as long as I could remember.

From that night on, I felt something change inside me. A tiny, almost imperceptible shift, which I know now must have been hope. I made running playlists, full of aggressive and fast music to encourage me on. I read running forums, amazed at those casual posts about people running twenty miles for fun. I browsed running trainers online before retreating, over-whelmed by the colourful choice.

Meanwhile, I laced up my crappy old pair every night and headed out. And every time, I went a little bit further. My lungs burned, and my shins hurt and I hated every minute but I was hitting ten minutes at a time within a week. Sheer stubbornness was powering me on. I would not roll over and give up. I would do it, even if I didn't know why I was doing it.

According to research undertaken by a team at University College London, it takes an average of sixty-six days to pick up a new habit and make it stick.[70] This requires you to repeat an action consistently, and within the same environment. Strictly speaking, I don't think running can be called a habit, but I was unwittingly using these guidelines to try to make my new activity take. And these sixty-six days might be helpful for you if you want to take up running, because so often I hear people say immediately that 'they hate running'. I used to say this too, but, since I'd never actually done it, it was a weak excuse. You don't hate running. You find it boring, or uncomfortable, or cold. But all of these things can be fixed, with time, form and equipment. Sixty-six days should see you right . . .

In the second week of alleyway running, my legs started to burn. Every time my foot landed on the ground, shooting pain surged up my lower legs, and I winced for the whole run. Maybe this was how running was supposed to feel, I wondered. Maybe it was a sign of my progress? Obviously it was not. A quick google revealed I had shin splints. This probably happened because I was wearing unsuitable gym shoes which had sat in a cupboard for eight years, or because

I was running too fast, and not striking properly. I still don't know if I strike properly, by the way, but I wasn't about to stop going because my bloody shins hurt. I gave in, and went to a specialist running shop. These places are ridiculously intimidating when you first go through their doors. They have lean mannequins in tight leggings and adverts for energy drinks and about 8 million shoes for different types of running, and I almost turned around and left straight away when I saw an actual TREADMILL in the corner on which you are filmed while they try and see what shoe you need. But I stayed, and lumbered away on the machine, and came home with neon trainers which cost a laughable amount. I'd put money in my running experiment. I was invested now.

The writer Charlie Brooker wrote about taking up running a few years ago.[71] He too had the intimidating-trainer moment – where you realise you're either in or you're out. 'I finally snapped and bought a decent pair of running shoes to replace the crappy trainers I'd been using. Once that dam was broken, I bought some wanky running shorts. Not one pair – but several . . . I can scarcely bear to look at myself in the mirror.'

Armed (footed?) with the proper shoes, I waited for the shin splints to ease up, and went back out there. Every time I wanted to go back home, I bargained for another ten seconds. Every time I felt nervous on a new road, I'd tell myself that I could always double back. And so, I started to edge out into the world. If, previously, I couldn't make it to my local high street because I'd start panicking, now I was jogging down it. I found myself exploring my neighbourhood anew – I marvelled at a bridge I'd never noticed, saw a collection of alms houses that were hidden down a lane. I started noticing familiar faces – the group of mothers with buggies in the local cafe; the man who drinks cider outside the fire station; the rug shop owner who carefully repairs his wares on the pavement outside. After years of wallowing inside my head, I was facing outwards. Running was allowing me to take a break from worrying. When I was busy concentrating so hard on not falling over, or not careering into an old lady with a shopping trolley, I had no time to panic.

And even in moments when I did feel the old familiar signs of anxiety creeping in, the physical act of jogging meant they couldn't get traction. The rhythmic motion – legs striding, arms swaying – becomes so regular that it can start to feel soothing. Side to side my arms went. One foot, the other foot. Body tilting. It was hypnotising. Breathing, which I was so used to being conscious of, was automatic. Breath in, breath out. Keep it going, even when it hurts. I needed the oxygen to continue, and that meant I had no time to worry about whether I *could* breathe, or whether my throat was constricting. I got tougher with myself. A twinge, or a surge of adrenaline, or a bad thought: I wouldn't entertain them when I was running. They had all my waking hours, but not these few minutes every day.

One month on from my husband walking out the door, I had cried buckets, I had drunk whatever wine I could get my hands on, I had smoked enough cigarettes to age me a decade and I had run further than I had ever thought I could. I had run in torrential rain, and in the dark, and I'd run when I was drunk, tired, weepy or furious. Sometimes all at once. I'd bought the trainers and I'd downloaded a running tracker. For the first time in a long time, I felt in control of something, however small. I didn't need to rely on anyone else to run, and I didn't feel like a feeble wreck when I did it. I didn't know it yet, but I had successfully formed a habit. I was hooked.

5K — EXERCISE IS
INTIMIDATING

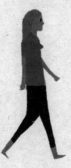

This is my second run of the day and neither of them have felt good. Not running to anything; running away; hoping the run will overtake my emotions and give me a break. Just eight months after a crappy turn of events had prompted me to start running, something immeasurably worse has happened. A family friend has died. But the term 'family friend' is an insipid, emotionless term. How do you describe someone who called herself your second mother; who gave you opportunities; yelled at you when you messed up; made you become an adult; and who would lock you in toilets until you told her good gossip? One of those individuals who really did make people turn around and say: 'Who is *that*? I want to know them.' While her death was expected after a long illness, it feels ridiculous that George, of all people, has gone. The space left is like the crater made by an asteroid – the hollow is scorched, deep and violent. So I am running all the time. In the morning, in the evening, whenever it gets too much and I think I will crumple. I'm not getting any high from it. In fact, I'm sweating because I'm going far too fast, hurting myself because it feels better than sitting and thinking about her. I don't want to let it sink in, so I run up Highgate Hill without stopping, until I'm forced to judder to a halt when I get a stitch. I sit on a bench in the dark and let my breathing return to normal. And then I carry on, because I don't want to go home and I don't want to cry. And because she was the toughest person I ever met, so I don't get to stop now. I don't yet know how to process such grief, but on this rainy night, running at least feels like an attempt.

You wouldn't be blamed for thinking that the appetite for exercise has surged in recent years. The innate desire to move has produced terrifying exercise tribes like the Tough Mudders, Barry's Bootcampers, the CrossFit Crew and the dedicated Spinners. Every week, a new regime is being breathlessly heralded as the best exercise you can do – a brilliant way to ward off obesity, osteoporosis, heart disease and depression. Some of it has an uncomfortable element of competition – a gentle stroll isn't enough, not when you could be biking twelve hours or doing yoga in a boiling-hot room.

But while records from Sport England show that 60 per cent of adults (27 million of us) do the recommended 150 minutes of exercise per week, a huge chunk (26 per cent) of us do less than thirty minutes of activity in the same period.[72]

None of this is helped by austerity measures which have had a helping hand in the decision to shut hundreds of play-grounds since 2014. Similarly, local councils have responded to budget cuts by closing public swimming pools and reducing other sporting facilities. And it makes a difference. Studies show that participation in sport drops noticeably in times of austerity. Where do you go to move if your local park is no longer maintained and grows neglected, or worse, becomes dangerous? This is not me being overly dramatic: in 2017, the House of Commons' Communities and Local Government Committee described UK parks as 'being at a tipping point', saying that 'if the value of parks and their potential contribution are not recognised, then the consequences could be severe.'[73] Not everybody has the money or time to go to a gym. We certainly don't make it easy for people to get up and move – despite all the official advice telling us just how important it is that we do.

It's not just limited resources that might put people off exercising, or the often exorbitant rates of private gyms – I sometimes worry about whether the perception of activity has been warped, turning people off the whole idea. It increasingly feels to me that, in the UK at least, exercise has been gentrified. While sport used to be seen as a pretty manly pursuit – featuring mud, testosterone and pain (off-putting in itself) – the modern image of a person who works out seems to have gone in a whole different direction, one which excludes just as many of us. Dispiritingly, I feel like pictures of those participating in exercise now usually end up showing sleek, glossy, rich white people. Instagram and other social networks don't help this perception – photos of slim women with visible abs or of men with rippling biceps don't usually inspire so much as alienate. It's no longer seen as enough to go for a quick swim at the local pool (I mean, of course it is in a sane world); instead you must join a gym which boasts its own nutrition line and pushes a confusing protein-shake regime.

Elite classes offered by SoulCycle, Barry's Bootcamp and CrossFit have long been popular in the USA, and they're on the rise in the UK, with sessions costing as much as £40 at some high-demand spots. And it's not just the type of exercise you take on which you are judged now, either: the rise in popularity of athleisure wear means donning workout gear which costs more than your normal attire – promising silver thread, moisture-wicking and extra speed. On one occasion I was almost tempted by a pair of leggings which promised to dissolve my cellulite as I ran. Do they work? Let me know. (I'm kidding, I know they don't work.) Every high street shop worth its salt now carries a sleek exercise-wear range, just in case you assumed it was acceptable to sport an old T-shirt and a pair of sagging leggings to work out in.

This image overhaul for exercise has pretty much gone hand in hand with the now well-established 'clean eating' trend, which encouraged people to cut out previous staples like sugar, gluten and processed food. The movement garnered so much criticism for its duff science and unhealthy approach that the practitioners quickly moved on to talking about 'wellness' instead. A much vaguer term, seemingly about intuitively listening to what your body needs, but still strangely doled out by the same impossibly thin, glowing and smiley posh girls who warned you off eating pasta. The whole crew of them ostensibly preached a 'no judgement' attitude where everything was allowed, but the message which seemed to cut through (for me at least) was one of deprivation, one-upmanship and physical image.

Forget the fitness and fashion magazines of yore, which you could easily avoid reading if you were concerned about unreasonable body expectations. Social media, which nearly all of us use to varying degrees, is awash with able-bodied beautiful people taking gym selfies, bragging about their abs, or filming their weight sessions. Just as I felt intimidated and unwanted by exercise as a teenager, I suspect a lot of these new exercise trends and images put people right off trying out any kind of movement. If you don't think you're the right size, or you don't have the money for £30-quid classes, where do you begin? And if your fitness level hovers around zero, as mine did a few years back, it can be easier to convince yourself that you just aren't made to do it. Those people aren't your people, so don't even try.

Every time I look at Instagram, even if I've just done a great run and feel all buzzy, I feel slightly dispirited by the sight of some lithe and gorgeous woman lifting her own body weight, or flashing her abs under the guise of showing off her breakfast. It looks too effortless, too smiley, too smug. And I'm not even exercising for a six-pack, so it shouldn't faze me. But that's now how easy it is to get you down or make you feel you're not trying hard enough. In 2017, the Royal Society for Public Health surveyed 1500 14–24-year-olds, and found that four-fifths of the most popular social media platforms were detrimental to mental health. [74] Instagram was the most damaging, presumably because photos are an effective way to show off and make others feel inadequate. This supposition is backed up by a 2016 study which found that people who looked at 'fitspiration' images on Instagram tended to feel more self-critical after viewing.[75] What an obvious but crappy finding. We are intimidated and disheartened by those who profess to inspire with their bodies. But of course we are – our bodies no longer stack up. How can they, when what we see is so filtered, so toned, so widely unachievable?

Marianne told me that she used to compete for her county as a teenager, but as she grew older, she felt increasingly uneasy with her body. 'I was increasingly unsure about what I wanted it to look like or whether the pain it was causing me was normal. I stopped exercising altogether. It became too painful to engage with myself as an embodied being. The absence of a mainstream societal story or image in which I could locate myself and which I might utilise in order to make sense of my experiences has massively, massively put me off exercising.'

Rightly or wrongly, the group of people mainstream exercise seems to cater for can seem too narrow for some people. Marianne saw what was on offer as unhelpfully divided down binary lines. 'Often it feels like one is either exercising "as a woman (sexed)" or "as a man (sexed)"; I'm doing lady-exercises and wearing lady-clothes as I do it and showing off my lady-body in a particularly nice Adidas sports bra. For people who have biologically female bodies, exercise clothing is limited to being skin tight and minimal in form. If one's experience of one's body is traumatic by virtue of simply being in one's body, then getting to the point where I feel able to even get dressed in order to go and exercise is often a bit of a push (and that's without the added complications of mental illness).'

We're letting people like Marianne down, and this is a crying shame. Because everyone lucky enough to be able-bodied should be moving more. Maybe more than ever before, we all need to be fitter. To prevent heart disease, diabetes, even to possibly ward off dementia. One in four of us is obese, according to the UN Food and Agriculture Organisation, and such figures are closely linked to social deprivation.[76] Statistics like these should be enough to get people up and out there, but seemingly they're not. And by the way, of course you can be overweight and exercise. Millions do – and for many, the purpose is not to lose weight. But these people are rarely featured in positive advertising campaigns or feted by our image-conscious culture. Nicola, a plus-size long-distance runner, tells me that she gets fed up when people 'look at me like I'm crazy when I mention I run. No wonder people are scared to start.'

Fed up with the lack of an inclusive and welcoming space in which to be fit and healthy, the body-positive movement has stepped in. The initiative, which came from the fat-acceptance movement of the 1960s, and was cemented by Connie Sobczak and Deb Burgard in the 1990s, endeavours to be inclusive, diverse and intersectional – celebrating bodies which have not always been accepted or praised by society. One of its aims is to promote the message that fitness should be about pleasure and fun, not about punishment or weight loss. If that sounds like something you'd be interested in, there is a good website which shows you where your nearest body-positive fitness teacher is – and the range is wide: yoga, boxing, whatever you think sounds fun. The website is listed at the back of the book.

So the image of fitness – privileged, expensive, undiverse and unattainable – needs to change. Because even without the physical benefits that exercise provides, which we're all aware of, exercise can give you a stonking mental boost – is that hammered home enough? It should be. Maybe more of us would try it if we knew it could help our minds and not just our hearts. Maybe more of us would do it if we didn't find it so intimidating.

I was pretty overweight at some points in my twenties, and I certainly didn't see a clear path to fitness. When I couldn't even wear clothes from high-street shops, I was unlikely to be seduced by the image that I saw the fitness market offering up. In fact, I was repelled by the honed bodies I saw around me. I saw no path to becoming like that, and missed any emphasis on feeling better rather than simply looking better. It was too intimidating. None of these smiley blonde fitness stars looked like me. Or even half of me. I was heavy, and uncomfortable, and ashamed of it. Not so much because I was big, but because I knew my shape was seen by many others as indulgent, lazy and unattractive. This didn't help any with my feelings of depression or low confidence. Exercise was about the body, and that felt like an area with which I wasn't familiar.

It's not just the overweight who might feel excluded. A 2015 study suggested that one reason the UK BAME population exercised less than the white population was because of a feeling that sport did not cater to their needs.[77] South Asian women, for example, reported a fear of racial discrimination at places offering classes or group exercise. Those of Islamic faith worried about the appropriate clothing needed, and whether the exercise on offer was for both men and women in the same group. Running is not exempt from this charge. Through his role, Alex Eagle (founder of The Running Charity) told me that he believes 'running is not seen as accessible to many BAME groups – it's [seen as] a traditional middle-class white sport.'

Asian and black women have the lowest participation in sport and exercise when compared to white women. And research in the USA shows that this starts early: physical activity drops hugely during adolescence, more so for girls than boys, and especially for ethnic minorities and girls from lower-income backgrounds.[78] A 2014 review of research into what prevented women (along with immigrants and underrepresented minorities in the USA and Europe) from underrepresented countries from exercising showed that responsibilities such as childcare and housework got in the way of participation. Cultural beliefs, social isolation, a dearth of culturally appropriate facilities and unsafe neighbourhood spaces were also noted as barriers to physical activity.[79]

At least part of that must be down to representation – who and what you see when you google a gym, or look up a sports kit, or see who represents the UK in international competitions – not to mention that the UK BAME population is also underrepresented in managerial positions and in sporting governing bodies.[80] To put it bluntly, people are being failed by a market which gives them no real thought. We must do better. Nobody should feel like they won't be welcomed by exercise, not when it's so vital to our wellbeing. That's why it was cheering to see the much praised Nike advert 'Nothing beats a Londoner' recently, which showed a diverse group of 258 locals playing sport in all areas of the city, in all weathers. More please.

For those with physical disabilities, the challenge can be even greater. According to a survey by Sport England, just 18 per cent of those with a disability or long-term limiting illness take part in sport each week.[81] Gyms can feel intimidating and inaccessible. But the NHS gives great tips on how to exercise with a physical disability, and the charity Scope can point you to a tool which advises you on which exercise will stand up to your specific needs. [82] The Activity Alliance (previously known as the English Federation of Disability in Sport) has a helpful section on their website which can help you find a local gym which will cater to your needs. [83] A link to their website is at the back of the book.

There are many reasons why people, especially women, might feel disinclined to try exercise. But as the 'This Girl

Can' campaign tries to show, sport isn't about being skinny, or living the lifestyle of a health nut. It's not even about being particularly good at your chosen exercise. It's about many other more fulfilling things. Physical health, mental health, a sense of achievement, a way to socialise, a time to relieve stress. As its research has shown, often we think that men have 'hobbies' which are positive, whereas women merely take 'me time', which is often dismissed as selfish or indulgent.

Exercise is something we're designed to do. Our muscles are made to be worked, our arms and legs (if we're fortunate and able-bodied) designed to move. But instead, we often view it as something totally distinct from us – either as worthy and merely to be endured, or elite and serious; and sometimes as a way to boost our bodies. We don't see it as an everyday task – like brushing our teeth. But we should.

I do it for my mental health, but that doesn't mean I don't appreciate the benefits that come with that – being able to walk up flights of stairs easily; eating a massive breakfast after a run; going out with my boyfriend to jog around the park when we're hungover. And it doesn't cost me anything, or require super-expensive kit, or demand I only eat soya and almonds.

I guess this could all sound a bit smug. Maybe it is, but I really don't mean for it to be – and please do bear in mind how little activity I did for the first thirty years of my life. It's only now that I exercise regularly that I see how tragic it is when people who can don't. How many years I wasted not giving myself and my body those endorphins, that rush, and that time. And sure, I'm biased, but it doesn't have to involve a complicated gym class with pulleys and weights – why reinvent the wheel when you can run, as our bodies are made to?

Recreational running has been around as long as we have.

People ran in ancient Egypt, in the Olympics 2700 years ago, and yet the practice fell out of fashion for much of history. [84] [85] As the writer and academic Vybarr Cregan-Reid, who wrote the brilliant book *Footnotes: How Running Makes Us Human*,[86] told me: 'Exercise emerges at crisis points in our history where there are forms of inequality. The Greek aristocracy invented forms of exercise because they realised they had to keep healthy for war, and then exercise sort of disappears for hundreds of years and re-emerges in the nineteenth century. Up until that point there are obviously people doing physical activity but there aren't people thinking, "Oh I need to get my steps in," because their day was their work.'

Professional sports people might have done it, but you weren't to see many amateurs out on the pavements in brightly coloured lycra. A turning point for the humble run came when a running coach called Bill Bowerman went to New Zealand in 1962 and was inspired by Arthur Lydiard, who had invented a running programme there. Back home in the USA, Bowerman wrote a pamphlet on the benefits of jogging for the non-athlete. The work was sponsored by the Oregon Heart Foundation, and popped up in Oregon banks. *The Jogger's Manual*, published in 1963, extolled the virtues of this new and exciting fitness trend.[87] 'Jogging,' the text explained, could be done 'anywhere' and by 'anyone – six to 106 – male or female'. Hilariously, it ended with the refrain, 'Good jogging to you!' I'm going to end this book with the same, obviously. On the back of this success, Bowerman wrote a bestselling book on the subject, and kick-started a trend. He tested his arguments on older subjects to show the benefits of running, and people listened. This work showed people that there was an easy(ish) way to develop a habit and shrug off a sedentary lifestyle.

Bowerman went on to collaborate with Nike, and the 1970s became a boom time for amateur runners. Since then, it's stayed a popular option for those casting around for a way to move more, and as a result, it's been the subject of numerous academic studies.

I'm *not* an academic, as many internet commenters have told me loudly over the years, and I can't begin to point you towards all the amazing in-depth research that has been done on exercise, particularly running, over the years. But I hope I can lead you to a tiny part of it, or at least show that my arguments in favour of running aren't fantastical. Results for many studies have been mixed, and it's worth pointing out that exercise can't help everyone who is in the grips of paralysing panic or sadness or grief. Nobody expects someone with severe and chronic depression to just get up and go for a run. It would be insensitive, unhelpful and pointless. In times when I've been laid up in bed, barely able to move, if someone had suggested a jog would make me feel better, I'd have stared blankly. Where would I have found the energy?

Indeed at least one study showed that exercise didn't help clinical depression,[88] perhaps because many people suffering from severe lows are also affected by psychomotor retardation – where your mind and body markedly slow down, giving you that horrible feeling of walking through treacle or having a woolly head. That would make it almost impossible to leap up and run. Instead, I think it's more helpful to see exercise as one tool in an arsenal. Something that can help, once you've got a foothold on the ladder out of the darkness.

Exercise has also often been seen as a way to *ward off* potential depression. The *American Journal of Psychiatry* did the biggest study of its kind on whether exercise can help with symptoms of depression.[89] Published in October 2017, the researchers surveyed 33,000 people with no symptoms of mental-health issues and found that those who did no activity were 44 per cent more likely to experience depression. In 12 per cent of cases, if the participants had done just one hour of exercise a week, the research suggested that depression could have been averted. So exercise actively protects against future depression, but unfortunately, the study did not say the same about anxiety. Bummer for me.

But wait! Research has also shown that anxiety sufferers *can* enjoy some mental-health benefits of exercise. Studies have shown a proven reduction in cortisol (the hormone released in response to fear or stress by the adrenal glands as part of the body's fight-or-flight mechanism) when people get up and move. In addition to physical changes, it's also been shown that exercise can change your thinking. In the book, *Exercise for Mood and Anxiety: Proven Strategies for Overcoming Depression and Enhancing Well-Being*, authors Jasper Smits and Michael Otto found that when anxious people exercised, they mimicked some of the symptoms of anxiety – fast heartbeat, sweat, adrenaline swirling – and that this actually made them less likely to panic when they experienced these feelings later on.[90] By associating them with something positive, the researchers suggested, people were not so scared of the symptoms. This makes sense to me – I no longer assume a heightened pulse is panic, and so the fear when I experience it has lessened.

Another study has thrown up a different reason why exercise might reduce anxiety, by studying stressed-out mice (imagining a stressed-out mouse is oddly harrowing).[91] This research, published in the the *Journal of Neuroscience*, showed that while exercise creates new and energetic brain cells, it also manages to shut them down when they're not useful. Two groups of mice were used in the control study – runners and sedentary. The runners were not only more confident and willing to explore their surroundings, but scientists found a number of new neurons present when they tested them – neurons which worked to quieten the brain. These were found in the hippocampus, the area associated with the processing of emotions. In effect, exercise was making the mice more resilient to stressful situations.

The neurons in the runner mice were producing more gamma-amino butyric acid (GABA), a neurotransmitter whose main role is reducing neuronal excitability throughout the nervous system. People with depression and anxiety can have lower levels of GABA, and research has shown that exercise fires up the pathways that replenish these neurotransmitters.

I've written all of this without even mentioning *the rush*. I have failed to sell running properly, I will go and apologise to my trainers. When I say rush I mean the tingly, euphoric bounce you can get from running. Hard to describe, and pretty fleeting. In the past, it has been commonly ascribed to endorphins – hormones released by the body. These little suckers interact with the receptors in your brain which reduce your levels of pain. Many experts initially thought this was why you got a 'runner's high' – a pale imitation of morphine, but a pretty brilliant non-druggy way to feel euphoric, ener-gised and bouncy.

This high might be hard-wired in humans. As Vybarr Cregan-Reid put it to me, 'The reason we have brains is because we move – the reason that plants don't have brains is because they can make their own food.' Back when our ancestors depended on catching their food (read animals, not a take-out on the couch), they did so with the knowledge that a failure to hunt meant death. David A. Raichlen, associate professor of anthropology at the University of Arizona, believes that the innate desire to survive was a pretty good motivation to go faster, and that the subsequent rush released may have helped them achieve the speed and distances required to get that food.[92] So exercise may actually make the body better able to respond to stress.

Newer research casts doubt on just how much endorphin production contributes to the runner's high. Some studies suggest that since endorphins can't pass from the blood to the brain (they're too big), serotonin (a chemical that nerve cells in the body produce) is more likely to be the reason you get a rush after exercise. Serotonin is one of four chemicals which affect our happiness – the others being dopamine, oxytocin and endorphins.

A 2012 study at the University of Arizona argued that anandamide (known as the Bliss Molecule) is a more likely cause of the runner's high, the rush we seek.[93] Sadly, anandamide (part of the endocannabinoid system), as with all other neurotransmitters, is fragile and breaks down quickly in the body, which is why we don't all walk around in a perpetual state of bliss.

Endocannabinoids, endorphins or serotonin. Or dopamine, or just the feeling of achievement, or even just the thought of going home and eating cake: I don't know what gives us the happy feelings that we get when we run, and I don't spend too much time worrying about it – as long as I can get it. I remember being very disconcerted when a psychiatrist first told me that nobody was 100 per cent certain why antidepressants worked, but I took them because I was at the end of my tether, and they worked. That's not to advocate blindly doing things that have no medical explanation behind them, but I believed that the drugs I took were safe, and I came to realise that they did what they said on the packet. Running for me is similar. There may one day be a conclusive answer as to why exercise makes us happier, and I'll read it with interest. But for now, I'll continue to do it, knowing that my sample size of one is testament enough for me.

And the high *is* real. We're no longer running miles to find our dinner (although I will happily run faster and longer if I know I can have a 99 Flake at the end of it), but the prospect of the rush still has a hold on us. It can be elusive – I have spent many runs waiting for it to take hold, but we're always chasing it.

I didn't feel it in my early jogs, when I was shuffling for mere minutes; nor in my later attempts, when I was running too fast and burning out, in pain and wheezing. But I would feel a bit brighter, a bit less tired, and I grew to like the tired feeling of having done something with my body. In her book about OCD, Bryony Gordon echoes this discovery – she began to run just 'to try and stay alive', and found that she always noticed that everything feels a 'smidgen more bearable than it did before a jog'.[94]

The first time I experienced a 'runner's high' was during a ten-minute session jogging down to Camden – a place normally on my no-no list, because of the crowds, the traffic and the panic I felt at getting stuck behind jostling tourists buying joss sticks and T-shirts. I had had a miserable week; sleeping on my own was horribly lonely, and I felt my adrenaline whoosh in the moment I woke up that Saturday and prepared to jog. But to my surprise, as I reached Camden, I felt suddenly springy. I didn't want to turn around and flee home where I would both reach safety and get to stop running. I wanted to push on. So I cut through the tourists and their selfie sticks, and headed down the canal.

By this point, the high had completely taken over, as I fairly raced down the path, wiggling my hands and bopping my head to 'Murder She Wrote', by Chaka Demus and Pliers, as far as I can recall. I remember grinning as I passed other runners, and marvelling at the beauty of the bridges I travelled under – places I'd seen a thousand times before, but never really noticed fully (one bridge is nicknamed 'the blow-up bridge', so-called because a passing gunpowder barge exploded in 1874, destroying the bridge, killing three crew and causing animals to escape from nearby London Zoo). I passed kayakers, which astonished me a little, and a boat carrying tourists down the canal, waving and taking photos. I discovered the Lisson Grove moorings, a community of houseboats which are surrounded by flower pots, hanging trinkets and wind chimes. It's utterly glorious. It feels like a secret neighbourhood in the middle of the city, hiding in plain sight but not much concerned with the land-bound goings-on above. I felt almost overwhelmed with how beautiful it looked, and stopped for a while, not wanting to ruin the ambience with an inelegant stumbled jog. I ended up at the final point on the canal before I was forced back onto the road by a huge blackboard someone had erected on the towpath. In huge letters, it asked you to write what you want to achieve before you die. Some people had taken it seriously, and spoke of falling in love and having babies. Some said they wanted to have great sex, and get drunk more. If I'd had any chalk (and if I didn't find it too cringe-making) I think I'd have written: not be scared.

That bouncy feeling stayed with me almost all day. Everything around me looked brighter, more welcoming, less sinister. I walked home in a happy daze, and didn't once mind the crowds humming around Camden Market, or the noise, or the traffic. I felt emboldened and as though I fitted right in with my surroundings. I felt normal. And I didn't get an anxiety stab in my stomach or start hyperventilating at all that weekend. Hell, I was even freed from my usual night terrors when I slept that night. See? Endorphins (or whatever it is). Magic; no wonder we literally chase that feeling down.

So while there are many valid reasons as to why so many people steer clear of exercise, there are just as many persuasive reasons why they should try and overcome these. But I probably wouldn't have listened to rational and (whisper it) dull arguments about why I should actively seek out sweat when I was younger. Maybe you come to it when it's crunch time. It will surely never stick if it's something you're forced to do, or made to feel guilty about. It's OK to find it on your own terms. But don't be like me, don't let the sometimes glossy perception of exercise make you feel as though you're not the right candidate.

If you want to move, and you're lucky enough to be able to, then you're the right candidate. That's all it takes. And sometimes, with some hard effort and a little luck, the misery around you might start to clear a bit. You might feel the relief that you've yearned for, and that we all deserve.

GK — PUSHING
THROUGH PANIC

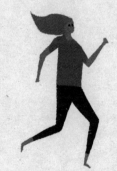

My first run abroad is in Venice. I have never much liked holidays as an adult. Too much to worry about in the build-up sort of ruins it for me. I missed out on so many trips in my twenties because I wouldn't fly . . . sometimes I have to try not to think about this in case I fall down a spiral of regret, which is pointless and unhelpful. It's more helpful if you see how far you've progressed. But yeah, I missed out on a lot of fun.

My mum decides to take me away for a long weekend, a respite after a year of grief and separation and general day-to-day life. My fears are all much quieter, after months of running and the weekly therapy sessions I am lucky to have, so I say yes, and this time with excitement. Venice is busier than I could've imagined, tourists shuffle past me with wheeled suitcases, looking at the ancient narrow alleyways with trepidation and awe. Others block the bridges so that they can raise their selfie sticks to the sky and capture the beauty (with their faces front and centre, of course). We eat and drink and walk miles up and down the Grand Canal, and after three days, I have a good sense of the city's layout. On our last morning, I'm feeling as relaxed as an anxious person can get – light, happy and ready to run. My mum is having a nap (my God does the woman love naps), so I head out across the railway bridge, dodging the latest travellers that the bus station has just unloaded. This is a run I never thought I'd take – I don't speak Italian well, I'm a stranger here and every main route offers up eighteen side streets and mini-canals for you to get lost down. I don't like getting lost usually – I panic and catastrophise about how I'll get home – but today, I let the route come to me, especially since I see I'll never be able to weave past the hordes effectively. So off I go down the first alley I see. People actually seem to live on this street – the city's population has fallen to 55,000 since a high of 175,000 after the Second World War – and colourful linens hang high above my head, slung across washing lines which zigzag between the buildings.

Venice doesn't instinctively feel like a place that welcomes runners, and I feel almost disrespectful to the historic buildings, but I pass at least three others who obviously know their route. If Venetians do it, then I'm probably OK. I try to run aimlessly and slowly. I have never seen such beauty in my life, and here I am, rushing past it all. Gondoliers push along deftly in the water beside me, and dogs seem to be everywhere – the locals love their small canine pals. By the time I stop to check the time, I'm completely lost on this small floating island, and I've done nearly 6k. A change of scenery and surrendering to my surroundings have pushed me on, and got me further than ever before. And nothing bad has happened! I feel strangely euphoric at being lost and not caring. Nobody knows where I am, and on the walk back to the hotel, I realise I don't want them to.

I'm writing this on the Tube. I'm on the Circle Line and we've been held up at Moorgate due to signal failures. So I'm writing to pass the time, getting used to a delay millions of people experience every day on London's overcrowded public transport system. It feels dull and fucking brilliant simultaneously. For me, it's not just a routine journey to be endured – I stopped getting the Tube on Millennium Eve. I gave my usual anxiety excuses about just preferring buses and not really caring much for the Tube, but really, I was shit scared of being under ground, being surrounded by people, of having no escape route.

I didn't get on it again for sixteen years and I lived in London the entire time. Nobody loves buses that much – especially in city traffic. But one day in 2016, I finished a long run some-where over the river. I had no more energy to head back on foot, so I loitered around the nearest Tube station. Could I? I must have stood there for nearly twenty minutes weighing it up. In the end, I compromised. I took a bus halfway and then swallowed my doubts and headed down the escalator to a windy and warm platform below ground. Buoyed by chocolate and running endorphins, I did the journey. It was all of four stops but I felt bursting with pride – even sending my family photos to prove it. It was one of the last stops on my list of things that anxiety had stopped me doing. One of the last things which made me feel like I was failing as a person. That and lifts, which used to scare me more than words, but now seem like a blessing when I have to go more than three floors. How strange, the things which stop us in our tracks for years, and become mundane, welcome, normal.

The tannoy is blaring out now. Signal failure means we all have to get off and now I'm wondering about getting the

Northern Line, which I still don't like much. Too deep below ground. But I'm working it out. I've learnt to celebrate any small victories and not berate myself too much if something is too hard one day. There will be another day when it's easier. Another run which helps me feel like I can do it.

Those little initial jogs I took, where I tentatively went down one new road before scurrying back, ended up leading to big messy routes, where I'd take a backpack and get lost in the city until I ran out of steam. No time for anxiety, no energy to engage with it. Someone once told me that they started exercising after coming across a quote, which I have, in vain, tried to find the author of. After much googling, I suspect it must be a play on something in Samuel Johnson's essay 'The Mischiefs of Total Idleness', but I like this better: 'Deep afflictions of the spirit are best alleviated by violent agitation of the body.' I'd like to have this written on a throw pillow. I don't know that I was violently agitating my body, but it certainly shook things up.

After I'd managed to run for about five minutes straight, I felt a bit lost. What now? For direction, I downloaded a Couch to 5K programme – you can find lots of these kinds of apps online, including one created by the NHS.[95] This programme gets you to run for a bit, walk for a bit, and builds up the running part until you can do it for thirty minutes straight (about 5km). If you're looking to start running, and feel like it's all an uphill battle, I'd give it a go. It's brilliantly simple and you can stay on the early levels as long as you want before proceeding to the next. You find yourself getting better at running, even as you tell yourself that you can't go on another step. The direction and order meant that even as I was covering new ground, I wasn't overwhelmed by fear or panic. I knew it would be one more minute ahead, one mile home. Nothing dramatic, just carefully planned distance. I put my faith in that programme, and by using it, I got to the holy 5k mark in six weeks. The day I finished it, it felt as though I was flying. Not in a spiritual way, it just initially felt like running for that long was about as possible as growing wings. I'd taught myself a new thing, and the satisfaction was immense.

Once I'd struggled through this programme, and struggle I did, I felt unleashed. I bought more trainers. I invested in good leggings which didn't fall down slowly as I jiggled. I bought numerous key holders and belts so that I wouldn't be weighed down with bags as I ran. All of this stuff was just frivolous merchandise, but it was a sign I was looking forward to something. Investing in trainers and water bottles was a silent promise to myself that I wouldn't stop, and that I'd acknowledged the good it was doing me.

And I really was looking forward to every run. Friends and family and work were all good distractions from everyday anxiety and marriage failings, but I wanted more. And I wanted to do it alone. So I kept on waking up early (my ex-husband hated my capacity to sleep the mornings away), forcing down a banana and heading out. Nowhere exciting – I chose main roads and flat terrain. I wasn't totally comfortable if I went somewhere alien, which meant I made a lot of repeat routes (if you're ever in London and in need of a run, I recommend the outer circle of Regent's Park: boring, repetitive, but manageable). None of these runs did bore me though, not really, despite the often mundane surroundings. I saw them as a chance to take little steps – going into a big shop I passed, or crossing a main road, or promising myself good coffee if I didn't wimp out and go home. 'Just one more minute' became my mantra. Anyone can do one minute, anyone can keep going even if they hate every second. Normally this meant at least five more, as I stubbornly refused to let my feet quit. And despite all my fears, I didn't have panic attacks, even as I ventured into unfamiliar places. I had silence, and space. Things an anxious mind is unfamiliar with.

As I grew more confident out on the streets, I pushed myself a little more. I had rational evidence that I'd be OK to go a little further, since I'd been testing out my limits, and finding them remarkably flexible. I looked up monuments, museums and historic buildings that I'd never visited and mapped my running routes around them. This often meant going through the busiest parts of town, where tourists dawdle and people rush about, where cars honk and everything sounds too loud. Things that I avoided like the plague. But when I was on foot, in a rhythm, using up all my excess adrenaline, it felt exciting instead of scary.

My first running adventure (adventure is probably too much of a sell, let's say jaunt) was to the site of Thomas Cromwell's house. I had recently finished reading Hilary Mantel's amazing *Wolf Hall* and had spent a lot of time googling more details of his life.

I found out he once lived on Austin Friars in the City of London, an area now famous for its glass-covered buildings and bankers in expensive suits. I looked up a vague route online and headed out. I had no idea how long the run would take me, so I ditched all plans for my Saturday. I started slowly, aware that whenever I'd kicked off running fast, I'd lost all energy within minutes. I shuffled down the Holloway Road, an arterial line running through north London, looking in the windows of old-fashioned hair salons, shops selling flashy phone covers and cafes where elderly ladies sat outside having coffee and cigarettes. I headed down Upper Street, past ridiculously fancy furniture shops and beautiful town houses with manicured hedges and blinds to keep snoopers like me from seeing their tasteful sitting rooms.

I was whizzing along now. Picking up the pace, listening to music as I wove through people walking along in the sunshine. I reached Farringdon, and the crowds thinned out. I passed an old fire station, a railway line and a centre for children who stutter. I ran through the old meat market in Smithfield, and stopped to see a beautiful church hidden away behind new buildings. I needed that stop, I was aching by now, and sweat was soaking through my top.

But I pushed on, running past St Paul's Cathedral, a place I hadn't visited since I was a child. There were bells ringing, and people gathering on the grand steps outside. Out of the corner of my eye, I noticed the Millennium Bridge – previously known as the wobbly bridge, which I hadn't crossed since its shaky early days. I decided to detour. I was feeling bouncy now, the runner's rush had kicked in and my legs weren't so tired all of a sudden. Off I went across the bridge, getting about halfway before I had to stop and look around me. I was almost smacked across the face by the beauty and grandeur of the city I lived in – a city I had been scared of for more than a decade. I had dreamed of escaping it, of living quietly in the country where I could avoid all the rush, the noise, the crowds and my own fear. But here I was, alone, standing on a bridge, seeing the city where I had been born in a new light. The city wasn't out to get me. It wasn't looming and cold, it was light and large and calm. The river ran underneath me, and for once, I wasn't thinking about the worst case scenario – the bridge collapsing and plunging me into the icy water.

I crossed over to the other side of London, and ran along to the next bridge – Southwark, where I returned to my previous route. On through the old part of London I went. The City is a magical secret place on weekends – all the bankers have gone home, and most of the shops are shut. The only people you encounter are vaguely bemused tourists who want to find the Tower of London. Every street has at least one blue plaque or historical sign telling you that you stand on the old site of Bedlam, or you are at the spot where the Great Fire of London started. Small historic buildings are squashed between the gleaming financial towers, stubbornly holding their ground. And the road names are nearly all another delightful reminder of another, ancient city – Pudding Lane, St Mary Axe, Bread Street, Ludgate Circus.

I got lost, and ran around a leafy square before I found Cromwell's road. Austin Friars, where he plotted and planned for (and sometimes against) Henry VIII. Only two parts of his house remain, and the Tesco just round the corner takes the historic edge off somewhat. But I was euphoric. I checked my running app (I use RunKeeper cos it's free and I'm cheap, but again, there are lots online – I list some at the back of this book), and I'd done 7k. The longest run I'd ever attempted, through parts of London I'd never seen, all on my own, with no panic. Nobody knew where I was (normally if I strayed away from home, I'd ring someone to talk to me so I wouldn't get anxious), and I felt light at this knowledge – I was my own master! I lingered, soaking up the feeling of freedom, feeling light on the knowledge that I had set out to explore a new place, and done it alone.

There is a section in *Wolf Hall* where Cromwell is schooling Henry, telling him blunt truths that nobody else would dare say to the King of England. He tells him not to go to war, that the expense will cripple him. The King says there must be more to his rule than prudence. Yes, says Cromwell, there must be fortitude. 'Fortitude . . . It means fixity of purpose. It means endurance. It means having the strength to live with what constrains you.'[96]

What a passage. No wonder it's become a slightly overused inspirational quote, often not even attributed to Mantel. I will never be a monarch, barring some huge constitutional upheaval, but that line came rushing back to me as I stood in Austin Friars. My first big run. My utter joy in holding back my anxieties to do it. I was living with what had constrained me my whole life, what else could I do now?

Running has taught me how not to be scared. From pounding the streets and tiring my brain out, my long-engrained phobias and fears about things like terrifying Tube journeys have gradually receded until they are just a fading bruise, and not a fresh injury. I know that my feet can take me places, and get me home too. I sometimes forget just how bound up I was before I started running, and writing it all down has been strange as I revisit just how miserable it all was. I recently went to see my wonderful former therapist, mainly because I missed chatting to him. He reminded me that when I'd first come to see him, just as my marriage was crumbling, I was barely able to leave the house. That low place seems far away now, even though I know that living with mental illness means never getting too complacent. I have anxious thoughts, and occasional nightmares and sometimes I get caught up in it all, but never when I'm running. It all goes away in those moments.

Starting something from scratch, and following it through,

was something I'd rarely been able to do before. That gave me a growing confidence, even early on in my running life. And that confidence gave me faith in my own body again. I was the route planner, the driver and the passenger. My brain had to shut up when I was busy deciding which road to go down, or when I was concentrating hard on getting my breathing even.

In effect, I was finally confronting my anxiety head on, and obviously it's not just running that can help you do that. But it's what I chose to try. If worry boxed me in, it seems natural that I chose to do something which afforded me an escape. But I still had to do more of what scared me, which was pretty much everything, really. It was a sort of exposure therapy – I was being dragged along by my worries until I had to dig my heels in and refuse to follow them anymore. Hiding from my fears had never worked, neither had engaging with irrational thoughts and arguing back. Avoidance is so tempting, but it's toxic – it reinforces the fear, and gives it strength. The panic balloons, spreads, engulfs you. Nevertheless, I always thought exposure therapy sounded crazy – the idea that you should confront the things that make you terrified. Why would you hold a tarantula if you're deathly afraid of spiders? But it's not as wacky as I imagined. This treatment took hold in the 1950s and involves a therapist exploring the origin of your fear, and what form the fear takes. It works particularly well on people with OCD or phobias. Say my mind works like this (and it does):

- A worry pops into my mind – e.g., what if this plane journey goes badly?
- I explore why I've had that thought and go straight to catastrophe – what if the plane crashes?

- I get the physical signs of anxiety – sweaty palms, heart palpitations, adrenaline, etc.
- These signs drum up more fear because they seem to validate the worry.
- Because I've scared myself so quickly, I start to panic.
- I don't fly on planes for five years to guard against the fear (that was fun – interrailing isn't so exciting when you're an adult, it's 40 degrees in your berth and you're sharing a bunk with a sweaty stranger).

As I've mentioned before, cognitive behavioural therapy encourages you to go back to the first question you asked yourself – what if this plane journey goes badly? – and then asks you to try and give the more rational and measured answer – e.g. the journey will be fine. A bit boring perhaps, and you won't have enough leg room. When you work through the questions like this, you slowly lower the fear response you produce when you run away with the catastrophic idea.

Exposure therapy is sort of similar, in that you are faced with, gradually, the thing or idea you're scared of, and hopefully the fear recedes as you realise that your worries are unfounded. It's maybe just a bit more dramatic.

You might be afraid of rats, and you could begin by saying the word over and over until you are comfortable with it. You might then look at a photo of the creature, and discuss how it makes you feel. Eventually, you might see a rat from a distance, or even touch one. God, even I don't really want to touch a rat.

For me, I did my own sort of exposure therapy. My threshold for fear is much lower than most people's. I'm not talking about pushing myself to do a skydive or climb a mountain here; my aims were tiny to most people. I wanted to go to see a friend by public transport and enjoy myself for an entire evening without worrying whether my flat was on fire, or if I might get run over, or whether my family were safe. I can do nights like that without thinking now, but I would never have been able to make them happen without running around first, learning that my fear wasn't always justified.

I pushed through fears that were etched into my being by putting on my trainers. I would identify a place or habit every day that gave me some level of fright – even if it was just a noticeably faster heartbeat. Just as with my short Tube journeys, I would force myself to run through crowded places – a market, rush hour, packed roads. And the catastrophes I had always suspected were lurking just around the corner never materialised. There were no panic attacks, no fainting fits, no bus crashes, terrorist attacks or typhoons or whatever else my mind sometimes threw up to make me stay at home, stay safe, stay small. If a route made me feel uneasy or jittery, I would do it again and again, until I was merely bored by it, rather than fearful or counting down the minutes until I could get home. Boredom is a strangely nice feeling after you've lived with excess adrenaline for so long.

If I felt particularly anxious or noticed my irrational thoughts bubbling up, I would force myself to run – even if it was just for five minutes. And there were a lot of days like that in the months following the collapse of my marriage. Sometimes, just the thought of going into work and seeing my estranged husband laughing with colleagues at his desk (which was a mere twenty feet away from mine) would send me into a spiral of worry when I woke up. Sometimes I felt like I couldn't handle another night sleeping alone, or face another evening where I saw nobody and sat in the silence of my empty flat. So I would go out and run before work, to shake off the adrenaline and be able to face the office. Or I would break up the long evening with a jog around the local park. And it would always calm me, always give me just enough strength to be able to go on.

It wasn't just the promised runner's high either. At this stage, I wasn't so much looking for a high as for a break. My mind would quieten down on a run, as though the part of it which tangles up my worries into knots, and gets stuck in a repetitive loop of intrusive thoughts, took a break while I was pushing along. It might have been put best by a runner called Monte Davis in Thaddeus Kostrubala's 1976 book *The Joy of Running*, who said: 'It's hard to run and feel sorry for yourself at the same time.'[97]

Because I probably did feel sorry for myself too much. I'd grown used to being angry with the world that I had this crippling worry. I'd ignored all the huge privileges I had been given – a loving family, financial security, a job, friends – and just focused on the one big problem I had. I blamed anxiety for holding me back, for ruining my marriage, for making me miss out on adventures, when really, I was letting it do all these things.

But running didn't make me angry. Frustrated sometimes, when I was out of breath or my feet felt like lead or I was too hungry to carry on further, but not raging. And the more I did it, the less wound up I would be when I had to deal with hard and uncomfortable moments. I could face them without running away immediately. When I found out my estranged husband was dating again, I felt like I would throw up, or fall down, or cry for days. But I didn't (well, I did cry for a short minute). I felt sad, and regretful about what was lost, but I also felt like I had an armour, however fragile, that now inured me to the worst pain. Not so much a shell, but a breastplate.

This felt like more than a thick skin – it was more like a new approach to life, where I wasn't fazed by the usual things so much. I was interested in whether I was alone in this feeling, and tried googling a few different terms – 'running makes me stronger', 'running makes me less emotional', 'running + no crying'. Eventually I stumbled upon a study from 2016 which looked into this very idea. Researchers asked half the participants to take a half-hour jog, while the other half did mild stretching. Afterwards, they all watched a moving clip from the 1979 film *The Champ* (YouTube commenters all attest that it 'demolishes' them). In those participants who had gone for a run but were prone to become emotional when faced with sad news or stressful situations, their usual negative reaction was subdued.[98] So I wasn't imagining my strange sensation of being armoured – aerobic exercise does seem to change the way people respond to their emotions.

And for those with busy brains, or who feel much more sensitive than other people, you can understand why running pulls them in. The legendary snooker player Ronnie O'Sullivan wrote an incredibly frank book about his addictions and anxiety. It's simply called *Running* – the thing he returned to again and again when he hit low points in his life (and he hit a lot, not least his dad going to prison for murder. You should read it, it's *a lot*). O'Sullivan writes about the 'chimp in his brain', which talks down to him and catastrophises (it sounds familiar, though I'd never anthropomorphised my thoughts before). These intrusive thoughts throw him off his game, and he works hard to push back against the addictions he's developed as coping mechanisms. And then he runs, and finds a way to beat back these negative ideas and habits. 'It had become an addiction,' he writes, 'but it was my best addiction yet by far. It's a continual high – one of those you can just repeat and repeat.'[99]

O'Sullivan lapses back into his old ways when he doesn't run. He writes again and again that he is a man of 'all or nothing'. I feel like this too. Moderation in anything has never seemed to fit well with me. I'm brutally miserable or bouncy and optimistic. I'm broke and worried or earning well and bountiful. And I can't take more than one day off running. Maybe it's a superstition – a compulsion like those weird tics I had as a child with OCD. If so, perhaps it's not healthy. Certainly friends have rolled their eyes at my insistence that I fit in a jog even on holiday. But I don't feel like it's unhelpful or controlling my life like anxiety has in the past. Instead, I bank on two things:

One: Running makes me feel less anxious every day that I do it. I never regret a run, no matter how much I don't want to do it on the day. I might well regret not going though, and that's a good thing to remember.

Two: I think it helps my defences against anxiety longer term. The science might be less clear cut on this than it is on point one, but I feel it for myself. Even if it's a mere placebo effect, that's OK with me.

From my long experience, one of the most important ways to deal with lifelong anxiety and/or depression is to accept that it'll be with you forever. It's a dangerous denial to hope or assume that you've coped with a low point well and must now be free of mental illness. The writer Eleanor Morgan, who wrote the excellent book *Anxiety for Beginners*,[100] put it well to me: 'There is no traditional happy ending. The happy ending is living with it.'

She's right. You most likely will never be 'cured' and become a different person who never experiences a symptom again. You understand that you have an illness, a disorder, a problem – whatever you like to call it, and you try to minimise it, and understand what might set it off.

Most importantly, you find tools to cope with it. And forcing myself to run every day, despite often not wanting to, works remarkably well for me. Six months after my big break-up, I contracted some kind of hideous tonsillitis which would not respond to any treatment the doctors threw at it (my mother insists the stress of everything had got to me and she's probably not wrong). Come Christmas Eve, a GP took one look in my mouth, and sent me straight to A&E, where I was promptly admitted overnight. Alone. On bloody Christmas Eve. After a bleak night of drips and jelly in a cup, I went home on Christmas Day and basically stayed in bed for two weeks. Illness always noticeably depresses my mood but the severity of this bout of illness meant I felt incredibly low. I cried a lot, and the intrusive thoughts started up again pretty fast. Like they had been preserved in aspic, they followed the same theme as years before – so much for having a nice change.

I learnt two important things from this episode, along with the worrying lesson that some antibiotics don't work for everyone. One was that every low moment didn't mean that I was spiralling back into anxiety and hysteria. Despite fearing a relapse at every turn, I also now knew that I had to look at

the facts rationally and reasonably. I was very ill, which naturally fucks with your brain chemicals, so feeling sad and worried
wasn't a huge surprise. It still happens when I get ill – my
mood dips and things stress me out more easily. Same with
hormones – the day before I get my period I invariably feel
extremely panicky and coiled up. But I know why it is now,
and that's half the battle. This is progress of sorts – I managed
to accept the low feelings without expecting them to usher in
another breakdown when I got very ill. I still have to do this;
my mind will always search for something looming, so it's
incumbent upon me to react with the more realistic scenario.
It's not always easy – my brain has usually done a few laps
around the track by the time I've realised I'm panicking and
attempt to push back. But you just have to keep doing it,
even when you secretly just want to lie down and allow the
anxious thoughts to take over. And that might sound perverse,
but when they've been your companion for life (and often felt
stronger than other emotions) it can feel like a relief. But it's
not. So push back. Keep pushing.

The second thing I realised was how quickly I bounced
back from this low. After glandular fever aged nineteen, I was
more depressed and anxious than I'd ever been before (in fact
I'm sure it was some kind of trigger for the subsequent breakdown I had). It weakened every part of me, and my family
would later joke that I was very much made in the mould of
a Jane Austen character – prone to taking to my bed and
being generally 'too weak for the world'. This completely
ignores that Austen also wrote strong and healthy female
characters ridiculed for their love of exercise like Lizzie Bennet
but I DIGRESS. This damnable tonsillitis, although horrible,
didn't leave any lasting impact. I ran again precisely two weeks

later. Embarrassingly slowly – almost back to square one, but I did it. And my body remembered doing it. I wouldn't say it was muscle memory, but it felt like a welcome return, and it wiped out the creeping worry I'd felt returning. Eleanor Morgan told me she experienced something similar after a serious surgery – a slump in emotion, a level of anxiety that only getting back to exercise could quieten again.

By then, I was feeling less raw about the break-up. Everyone I knew was now fully cognisant that my husband had walked out within a year of our marriage. There were no more reactions to brace for, no sad looks or tilted heads of sympathy. I was somewhere on the road away from heartbreak, feeling OK. I'd even been on some fairly dismal dates. So I wasn't great, but I was better. And this is what I know to be a dangerous place for me to be. Just when my anxiety is less, when I feel pretty stable – that's often when I stop trying to keep it like that. I get complacent and think I've cracked it. But as Eleanor Morgan said – you have to live with it. If I hadn't become ill and had the experience of a temporary slump, I suspect I might have given up the running. I felt like I'd cracked it, I felt it had been helpful. Did I want to run marathons and do cheery park runs and worry about personal bests? Did I really want to do it forever? I didn't think so, but realising I wasn't rid of anxiety that Christmas doubled my running resolve. I'd finally found a way to help myself, and it'd been hard won. I'd have preferred my salvation to come in the form of wine and a sun lounger, but life is pain, and anyone who tells you different is selling something.*

---

* If you don't know this quote go and watch *The Princess Bride* immediately. You're welcome.

7K — WHY DO WE RUN?

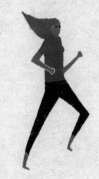

I ran around Edinburgh today. Leaving my friend and my phone at the hotel, I decided to wing it. I set off direction-less down the main shopping street, gawping at the castle, which was bathed in red light. Cobbles felt wobbly under my feet and I could sense my ankles were in danger of rolling. But I focused on the road, and got into a rhythm. This was the first run without my phone – my safety net. I'd never even been to the shops without it – just in case, just in case, just in case of what? I didn't know the city, and normally that would have made me more nervous, but today I felt freed by that knowledge. I was all alone and it felt fine. Maybe more than fine. I felt giddy abandon. Edinburgh is hilly, and my lungs protested by burning as I went, but the beauty of the place strengthened my resolve. I found a road which seemed to promise a gentler pace, and swerved off the main stretch. After half an hour, I found myself in Leith, the port district in the north of the city. Everything was quieter out here, and I could see seagulls buffeting on the winds in the distance. I decided they were the way to the water, and I tried to track their movements as I ran. I rounded a corner and came upon the docks, screeching gulls and all, and gasped. In front of me was a ship painted in glorious technicolour – a 'Dazzle' ship, designed to commemorate the Battle of Jutland. These brightly painted vessels originated during the First World War, and were covered in disorientating shapes and bright colours to prevent the enemy from figuring out their speed or direction of travel. The artist who designed this one named it *Every Woman*, as a tribute to those who helped create the original Dazzle ships. It's glorious and mesmerising, every line and curve feels like a tribute to strength and resilience. I stood and stared at it for longer than I meant to, wanting to absorb those things, wanting to keep it in my mind.

On the way back, I tracked down the royal yacht *Britannia*, which is considerably less grand, with access to it found through a shopping centre – the lack of majesty here amused me so much I got the giggles and for a moment I didn't feel I could run home.


Why do people decide to run? I'm not talking about the brilliant early adopters who picked up sports at school and continued to make time for physical activity into adulthood. I am in awe of those people but I'll never be like them. I left exercise for decades, often resent it, and only still do it because I have to grudgingly admit how much good it does me. Those people always knew how good exercise was for them. They might say it's just a part of everyday life, like lunch, or having your card declined (just nod and reassure me). I wonder why people run when they don't have this mindset. When they've sat on couches for decades, when they've driven to the corner shop, and waited for another bus rather than leg it and break a sweat. I've talked about how, as kids, we expend so much energy running about.

I believe it's in our nature to stretch our legs and career about, but we forget this as we grow up. It can easily be buried forever, so how come some of us return to it?

Physical health is obviously a big draw – running can help keep your weight under control, improve cardiovascular fitness, limit your risk of diabetes. As Vybarr Cregan-Reid told me, 'Our body rewards us for movement – it makes us tougher, stronger, makes our bones thicker, helps with serotonin, nor-epinephrine and dopamine. It gives us the means to be more intelligent.' A study in America found that an hour of running can add up to seven hours to your life – even if you have bad habits like drinking and smoking. Good news for me. But then, walking, swimming and many other activities are also proven to be good for you. And you don't need to see January joggers to know that many people give it up almost as soon as they start it. Over 20 million Brits are said to be inactive, according to the British Heart Foundation.[101] We seem to have forgotten that our bodies need to be used. Despite the constant campaigns to let us know about the health benefits of exercise, the reasons people get up and move don't always seem to be about basic fitness.

Instead, when it comes to running, it often seems that a crisis kick-starts our urge – or reveals it after years of it lying dormant. Maybe it's just a need to get away from our problems as fast as possible, but I think there's much more to it. The modern world means being sedentary and inside of our own heads most of the time. We're used to this by now, grateful we don't have to toil in fields all day, and that we instead get to surf Facebook in a heated office while we're meant to be working. But at times when we encounter ruptures to this comfortable life, it can suddenly not feel like enough anymore. We no longer wear ourselves out physically, and that is, understandably, acknowledged as progress. The disconnect from our own bodies has become the norm, since many of us no longer live lives which demand that we exert them. But sometimes, the comfort we've allowed ourselves is no longer enough, and a hard day makes you want to get up and scream, or throw something across a room, or rip off your clothes and beat your chest. Life stifles you and you seek to break it open dramatically. You don't, because you don't want to be an embarrassing YouTube moment for the rest of time. So maybe you search for something which gives you a similar feeling of relief, where you can shrug off the worry and the monotony. Where you can do something hard – something which matches how hard life is at times. And that's often when I think people find running.

The Tibetan Lama Sakyong Mipham is the leader of a meditation community. He also loves to run. To Mipham, the two things enable each other. I picked up his book once at a particularly low point several years ago, wondering if I was missing an element to my running – should I be feeling more deeply when I run, am I missing something powerful? Yet as I read *Running with the Mind of Meditation*, I realised that much of what the Lama said I had already (albeit uncon- sciously) experienced. 'Just as in running,' he writes, 'in meditation we leave behind our daily concerns – the daydreaming, stress and planning. By doing that, our mind builds strength.'[102]

Stephen (not his real name), told me how a mixture of mindfulness and running dug him out of the anxiety and subsequent depression he had struggled with since childhood. 'I've always been anxious,' he said. 'My parents had an acri- monious break-up and my home life wasn't great. I first experienced depression aged seventeen, and left school early. I'd gone to an exam and written nothing for two hours. I walked out. Before that I'd been an A student.'

Steve got into university a year later and had a great time. 'Distraction activities,' he told me. He later went into computer work and had a family. Now 56, Steve was diagnosed with depression ten years ago but says, 'I reckon I must've been depressed for quite a while before that. My behaviour became bad. My mind was whirring and I'd snap at my family, and bring down the mood of my whole house. I had some counselling through a work programme but I didn't find that it helped.

'I couldn't quieten my mind . . . There was no relenting . . . and then of course if I got edgy and snapped at someone that would contribute. It was a feedback loop. And then you start disconnecting from things. I was unable to function, not doing anything good for the family and shutting off.'

Eventually Steve went to see his GP and almost cried in the surgery. 'They slapped me on Prozac and told me I was quite severely depressed. I felt very nervous about taking it and I thought, oh my God, this is something affecting my brain.' But Steve took the prescription and found that 'two to three weeks later it (the depression) just lifted. I felt human again. It gave me the impetus to say, right, counselling didn't help, what shall I do?'

A friend who ran signed Steve up to do a 10k. He did it, and then signed up to do a marathon. And then another. Alongside this, Steve found an experimental mindfulness programme, and discovered that the techniques it taught him worked in tandem with his running. 'Running is mindful for me, because I think a bit, I'm looking out for things and noticing the seasons, or I listen to what my legs are saying.'

Steve now runs long distances with a running club, which he credits with maintaining social contact (he works away from home a lot). 'The running and the ability to calm my mind with mindfulness techniques meant I felt I could come off the Prozac. In the last year I've taken up singing too. Those are now my three supports.'

As I've done with everyone I've spoken to for this book, I asked Steve what running makes him feel. It's a question which always gives new answers, and Steve's made me smile. 'Anticipation and wondering how a run is going to go beforehand. Once I've done two or three miles the engine will start, and then it's pleasurable. I get an almost childlike joy when I run fast downhill.'

That childlike joy is a brilliant tonic for the weights we collect as we go through life. We all need to leave behind our daily stresses at some point. We need balance – when we stay on the daily treadmill, our minds buzz and bleep and we get bogged down in the immediate. We don't often actually take those important breaks though – at least not willingly. But life often intervenes and makes us, whether we want to or not.

Out of all the life ruptures human beings experience, a big break-up like mine is probably the most common. But there is also grief, mental illness, job loss and others more cheerful but no less challenging – like becoming a parent or moving across the globe. I spoke to so many people during the writing of this book, mainly to ask them why they started running. The answers were revealing, but honestly? Never really surprising. The stories were different, the difficulties broad in scope, but everyone who told me their story had a common desire – to try to find a way of escape. To ease pain, and to lessen hurt. To take back a semblance of control.

Let's start with love affairs which have gone wrong. This may be selfish because it's where I started, but it's my book so just humour me. Those of us who haven't experienced rejection or disappointment in relationships are few and far between. I wouldn't even call those who avoid it lucky. It gives you a life lesson you have to learn sooner or later, and a partnership which fails can be instrumental in showing you what you *don't* want in any subsequent relationships you might have.

Heartbreak can make even the most well-balanced people veer off kilter, so of course it has the power to make those with mental-health problems feel so much worse. When everything around you feels out of your control, it's easy to understand how people seek out something which they can exert some semblance of choice over. Remember that for those with anxiety, the fear of losing control is immense. And there's nothing like a relationship breakdown to make you feel you've lost all your autonomy over your emotions.

Peter had a similar urge to get out and run when a big relationship went south. It left him reeling, and provoked negative feelings that he'd never had before.

'I fell in love with my best friend of eight years. She waited until I moved from Dublin to Toronto to tell me that she loved me. When I moved back eighteen months later, I realised I couldn't shake my feelings for her. So I told her I was in love with her. I moved to London to be with her immediately.

'Naturally it didn't last because we never came up for air. After we broke up I moved out and was at a complete loss. I had no idea what to do with my life on any level. I left

London and moved back to Dublin into my parents' house.
I did nothing for six months except exercise and complete
crosswords.

'I had no idea I was even depressed. It kind of crept up on
me. I mean, how are you supposed to know you are depressed?
With the benefit of hindsight, I can look back now and
acknowledge that I don't ever remember feeling even the tiniest
moment of happiness during those six months.'

Not knowing you've got a problem while you're in the
middle of a mental-health crisis is very common. It can be
hard to see the wood from the trees when you're in the depths
of sadness. Peter says he looks back at photos from that time
and, again with the benefit of hindsight, sees the huge black
rings under his eyes. Despite this, he started running five miles
a day (I am still in awe that he managed to do this much
when he was feeling so terrible).

'My head and thoughts were completely empty when I was
running. I wasn't over-analysing anything or worrying or
feeling sad. I knew I had five miles to run every day and it
was an achievable goal. With everything else completely going
against me (which might not have been true but it felt like
it), I knew I could run five miles and not fail. The only thing
that held me together was running, so I could physically clear
my head and stay in shape, and crosswords, so I could keep
my brain working.'

Peter also mentions feeling completely at a loss, so the target
of five miles a day tethered him to something, and gave him
back that much prized control.

'Setting myself an achievable goal meant I had some
semblance of control over my life, because it felt like I was
absolutely lost in an ocean where I was swimming against the

current in every single direction. This was one tiny area I could control; get out of bed and sprint for five miles.'

Peter's urge to set a small goal and stick to it echoes my initial running motivation entirely. A more recent personal setback had him back out pounding the pavements again. And as it had before, running has given him the resilience to cope with new sadness and disappointment. 'Everything comes back to running when stuff happens to me; it's the only thing I can control at the time because my emotions are all over the place and I am unable to get a grasp on them. Control seems to be the theme.'

Seeking control can often sound like a negative thing – an unhealthy need to be in charge, or a rigidity which precludes spontaneity. But when you're miserable, I think it's just a desperate desire not to feel like you're in freefall with nothing to grab onto.

My running started at a point when I felt I had no say in what was happening in my life. My husband had left, and I couldn't shake off the increasingly anxious feelings that I knew at some point would consume me totally. Forgive the bad analogy, but my life felt like a horse that had bolted away from me, and I was racing to grab the reins before I lost it forever. Running allowed me to feel like I was in touching distance of those reins.

Every time I managed to go a little further, or venture into a place I'd previously been scared of, I felt like I was chipping away at the shame and misery and panic that I was so used to. Heartbreak is a gut punch in so many ways, but the physical pangs were what I hated the most. Any thought of what I'd lost and I'd be curled up on the bed, or crying in the toilet. It's an immediate and surprising reaction – one that comes with nausea and trembling. It makes your body feel weak and your mind feel defeated. And it makes you want to retreat, even to wallow in that seductive place where darkness and bad poetry lurk.

But that's a trap – nobody ever feels energised and powerful after three hours of listening to the Smiths and looking at photos of an ex.

What works is pushing back against those moments of melancholy. I don't mean you should ignore your feelings and deny your sadness. A very clever therapist (Hi, Barry!) once told me that whatever emotion you're feeling at the time is the correct emotion for the time. Or something like that, I hope I'm not misquoting him (Sorry, Barry). But I've always remembered it. Sadness isn't something to worry about – you're feeling what you're supposed to be feeling. But you don't have to entertain it, invite it to stay longer and make up a bed for it.

I hated those gut-punch moments, when my immediate instinct was to retreat. I'd done enough retreating in my life. So I decided not to. I didn't want those feelings of loss and regret to be on my mind all the time, and believe me, they were. So if I got a burst of them, I'd force myself out for a run.

No time for nausea, no duvet available. Just a challenge, or a punishment, depending on how I felt on the day. Either way, it was something I had to see through. Someone had stopped loving me, and that rejection would drive me on in a way it couldn't or wouldn't in normal day-to-day life. Running managed to stifle mocking memories of wedding vows, of promises made, and also lessened the impact of remembering how it all went to shit so quickly afterwards. Even on days when I hated going out in the rain, or dragging myself out with a hangover, I knew I was giving myself something good, rather than entertaining my sadness. As I've said, the moment of heartbreak is brief, and then you have to go through the 'getting over it' process. Running provided an extra layer of defence against all the painful emotions that a relationship breakdown throws at you. Peter summed it up brilliantly: 'It doesn't make sense but I feel bulletproof and that I can handle anything.'

Some break-ups are worse than others. Mine was dramatic, surprising and embarrassing. But I got to the other side fairly fast in the end, unscathed and relieved. I was lucky; sometimes the grief at losing a partner can bring on serious depression and exacerbate anxiety.

Alva had a boyfriend who cheated on her. She stayed with him, but struggled with the heartache and became incredibly depressed. 'I didn't have any other explanation as to why to stay with him than I was scared. Scared to lose him because I loved him, scared to be lonely.'

Her depression escalated: 'I felt ashamed of struggling, I felt like people wouldn't understand. It made me unable to ask for help. My depression put me in the place where I would say horrible things, and I wouldn't be able to cope with myself and the surroundings.'

Eventually a suicide attempt put her in hospital and her boyfriend broke up with her when he realised that he had contributed to her unhappiness. Her doctor recommended she try exercise, and while she was sceptical, she gave it a go. 'I started off by walking shorter distances, then they became longer as my energy levels increased. Then they turned into shorter jogs and so it improved more and more. I didn't understand at first but eventually I could wrap my head around how nice it felt to be just as tired physically as I was mentally.

So I joined a gym and saw a poster about a 10k run. The feeling after passing the finish line was so good, a pleasure I hadn't felt for so long – and it made me want to continue. I wanted a bigger challenge though, so I signed up for a half marathon. I completed it and felt the exact same way, so I signed up for a full marathon this summer. I'm not saying that everyone should sign up for races, but for me it becomes a goal, which makes it easier for me to tie my shoes and make myself come out for a run.'

Alva now pushes herself with marathons, increasing the challenge and seeing how far she can get. I've never wanted to sign up for a race, though I completely understand the allure of seeing what your body can do. I've been happy to plod along regularly, and not at any speed. As Alva says, not everyone needs to do competitive runs – sometimes it can be intimidating to start running when you see ultra-fit people who can rack up the miles with ease. I've never thought I'd be a good long-distance runner (I get hungry stupidly fast), and I'm fine with it. You do what feels good for you – if that's a marathon, then fantastic. If it's a jog around the block when you're stuck in a fog of depression, then that's equally brilliant.

Now that she runs masterfully, Alva can describe her recovery from depression beautifully: 'I know that if someone had told me their story and explained how running helped them, my condition wouldn't have been as bad and I wouldn't have let it go as far. Time has given me perspective though, and I've realised that I shouldn't be any more ashamed of feeling depressed or low than a person who has broken their leg and asks someone to hold the door for them.'

I spent years denying my anxiety and depressive episodes. I'd worry that people would treat me differently, judge me or back away from me. Even as I got older, I'd downplay my anxiety, joke about it, never tell anyone the dark thoughts that occupied my mind. 'I'm just feeling a bit down' was my common refrain, or I'd make excuses and cancel plans, leave places early, tell my boss I felt sick, rather than explain I couldn't get on the bus because I'd had a panic attack. I once had to sit down in the street because I thought I was dying, and when it didn't pass, I called an ambulance and went to hospital. I'm embarrassed now to have wasted NHS time and money, but it's a measure of just how bad I felt. I told work I'd fallen over, rather than admit I couldn't cope with what was going on in my head.

Alva told me her story freely because she wanted people to know it was OK to talk about it. Her recovery showed her that there was nothing to conceal, and no reason to feel embarrassed about telling it. It's often easier to talk about mental-health issues when you feel you've gotten over the worst of it – the skies have cleared somewhat and you no longer view yourself so negatively. Mental-health issues come with a huge amount of self-criticism, very rarely do people who struggle with these issues not blame themselves in some way, even fleetingly. I was no different, and it wasn't until I began to run that I felt I could talk to people more openly about how I had struggled over the years. It helped that my story made sense to people – a bad break-up had led me to try running, and that in turn allowed me to mention that I also had some anxiety issues that were worse than I might have let on. In a funny way, having a horrible relationship collapse meant I was open about my other issues for the first time in my life. Always a silver lining, huh?

Running has helped people through heartache – offering a

brief escape from the sadness, and the ice-cream eating, and the sad songs that Spotify just casually tosses up. But while a relationship split involves the loss of another, it's not the worst pain you can feel. As my mum might say, 'Nobody died.' Or as Stephen King said (and as featured on every inspirational Pinterest board): 'Hearts can break. Yes, hearts can break. Sometimes I think it would be better if we died when they did, but we don't.'[103]

But what if somebody does die? What if you experience grief so intense that you can't imagine anything coming close to comforting you or soothing the pain? When the writer Catriona Menzies-Pike lost both her parents in a plane crash in her twenties, she turned to running to attempt to deal with the loss. And this was not just casually jogging aimlessly when the mood took her, like I have often done – Menzies-Pike started doing long-distance runs. She suggests that the structure and discipline involved in training for a marathon provide the order that those who have lost everything are looking for. In her book *The Long Run: A Memoir of Loss and Life in Motion*, she explains: 'The aftermath of loss is exhausting, repetitious, and often very, very dull – and so is training for a marathon. But endurance can help turn elusive sorrows into something tangible, like aching muscles and blisters. Such pain can be easily described.'[104]

Antidepressants do not make you happy and running can't always give you a high. In times of utter sorrow, you might do it to punish your body, to make it physically experience the pain you're feeling mentally. Sometimes it can force you to focus on something other than your grief. At best, it might help numb the sadness somewhat.

Having started running to combat my rapidly worsening

mental health and push out the sadness of my break-up, I soon learnt that running couldn't insulate me from grief. But, just as it was helpful in calming my mind and providing me with the space to deal with my worries, it could also guide me through worse.

After several months of running, I was a firm convert. I felt better, I was no longer plagued by panic attacks or constant and obsessive thoughts. I could think about my husband without crying. I would bore people with this news, explaining how the high after a run could beat any drunken night out. And then my friend died. My mentor, my other mother.

George had been ill for a while, fighting aggressive cancer with her natural determination and core of steel. But it became clear early on that she was not going to be able to beat it (I hate that phrase actually, as though some people can win against cancer with their own will, and others can't). We spent a wonderful summer holiday with her, where she drank Negronis and lay on the lilo wearing a big hat and sunglasses, looking as glorious as ever. We spent New Year's with her, and she was much sicker, but she laughed as loud as ever as she mocked my dad and demanded gossip. And then she was suddenly and dramatically worse, and even though we knew it was coming, I didn't really believe it. How can you truly imagine the most energetic person you know not being in the world? It feels like physical space has gone wrong, as though our delicate existence has broken.

The day she died, I calmly left work and walked home. I wasn't overwhelmed with grief, because I genuinely couldn't picture her not being here anymore. I guess that's a classic delayed reaction, because I eventually did picture it, and then the grief was total.

The running I did after we lost George was all-punishing. I would run longer, faster, in the rain, uphill. I was running to push out sadness by inviting in physical hurt. Legs burning, lungs working overtime, heart pumping. I got no physical rush from it, no high and no sense of achievement. I just did it to do *something*.

At first, I wasn't entirely sure that it was helping at all. Unlike my early running, where I felt better immediately after a jog, and felt my negative feelings lift a little bit more each time, I didn't feel much relief. But the physical unpleasantness of hard runs slightly negated the mental stuff. And it seems I'm not alone in this 'putting pain on pain to feel better' strategy. In a 2017 paper by researchers from Cardiff University titled 'Selling Pain to the Saturated Self', the authors looked at people who completed a hard physical challenge – the Tough Mudder – to try and understand what pain does to us.[105] The Tough Mudder is a series of twenty-five brutal exercises – fancy running through a bog or risking electric shock? If so, this is the day out you want. The authors wanted to know why people would actively put themselves forward for this kind of pain, rather than run screaming from it like I would. From interviews with Tough Mudder participants, they found that physical discomfort seemed to suspend people's usual brain activity. 'When pain floods their consciousness, participants seem unable to develop complex thoughts. Pain temporarily suspends the reflexive project of the self.'

So by running, and feeling it in every part of my body, I was able to shut off the feelings of grief that had enveloped me. Not for long, and not forever, but enough to see some light. As the Cardiff study showed: 'Pain enables a temporary erasure of the self. When flooding individuals with unpleasantness, pain momentarily erases the burdens of identity and facilitates a distinctive type of escape.'

Erasing the burdens of identity just nails it, I think. Life is hard, the emotions we have to deal with can be too complex for us to handle. Sometimes you want to shrug off the hardships of being a human, if just for a few minutes. Going running is not an attempt to pretend life is *not* hard; it's a break, a lift, a pause. The researchers summed up their exploration of physical pain by saying: 'Escape is not always grandiose. Escape also lies in the ephemeral and unremarkable instants of dis-identification.'

Chris started running when he was faced with the impossibly awful news that both his parents were terminally ill. 'Dad had dementia, chronic obstructive pulmonary disease and lung cancer. Mum had motor neurone disease, and lost the power of speech. She was meant to be looking after Dad. It didn't work out well.'

In a bid to retain some semblance of control, Chris told me that he fell upon running. 'I couldn't help the situation much, beyond organising carers, hospitals and so on, but I definitely could make sure I took care of myself, and reduce the chances of me ending up in a similar position with my kids. Partly fear of that, probably. It also got me out of the house, so a constantly changing scenery helped put distance between me and my worries.'

Running with grief is different to everyday running, when you're chasing a high, or seeking a rush. Chris wanted to feel he could do something notable, at a time when he felt helpless. 'After the first run – which made me feel dreadful because I thought I was fitter than I was, and left me gasping while trying not to be sick – things gradually got better in terms of physical fitness, but I think I was hooked on the idea after about two or three runs. It wasn't the endorphin thing people talk about – although that might have played a part later – this was more a good feeling because I was being disciplined with myself. I started running in the evening, but after those first few I decided getting up earlier was better. Running at that time made me feel like I had achieved something even if the rest of the day was a shocker.'

Running helped Chris throughout this sad and stressful time in his life – both physically and mentally. 'It distracts you a bit because your body is doing something. I think that slows down parts of your mind, and if your lungs are bursting or your legs want to stop, other thoughts have to wait their turn. Only the really important things get thought about, so that helps you sort the wheat from the chaff. It prioritises things, and helps to organise thoughts. It also reminds you that you're human, particularly if you get out at dawn. That conjures up primeval images in my head, and reminds me of my place in the universe. Sometimes, you just don't think at all, and before you know it you've finished, but you're calm and mentally refreshed. What I'm trying to say is that, above all, it helps bring perspective.'

The energy that running gave him helped him deal with the day-to-day difficulties of caring for his mother and father, a stressful and demanding role which could quickly become exhausting. 'Being physically more capable helps deal with stress, I think. It can be a tiring, and a terribly draining thing, so having stamina certainly helps.'

Chris is quite right. Grief is exhausting. Stress is exhausting. Any reserves you have can fade away in a split second, and you likely don't take good enough care of yourself when you're busy caring for others. Running can give you back some of these reserves. It's not a massage, or a pedicure, but it's self-care all the same, and will give you more back than a blow-dry. For many, time for yourself is seen as an indulgence or a luxury, but it's neither – it's vital to recharge. Twenty minutes sweating outdoors is something powerful you can give yourself. Chris still runs three or four times a week, and called it a comforting 'old friend', which I *loved*. Highs and lows come and go, but running remains. 'You know it will help. I think other people have it a lot worse than me – I just had (have) some problems to deal with.'

And that's true of all of us who run, hoping to tackle problems and shrug off loss and sadness. A person might look like they're doing a casual 5k, but you can't possibly know why they are *actually* running past you, screwing up their face as they pound up a hill. It's a mundane everyday activity done by millions. But so many of them will be taking a mini-escape. Not a decision to run for the hills and never look back, but a way to willingly return to their life with a calmer mind, or a quieter brain. Running remains through it all.

While I firmly believe you have to find your own running sweet spot, and that it's important not to compare yourself to others, I'd also like to highlight the people who run races for another reason. The people who run marathons, races, park runs, all to help other people. Awful situations get people running, but they also inspire some to do good. You only have to look at charity runs to see how many people use exercise as a way to raise money and awareness for good causes. In 2017, the London Marathon collected £61.5 million for charity – bringing the total raised since the event began back in 1981 to over £890 million. In a sign of the times, the chosen charity that record-breaking year was Heads Together

– the charity founded by the royal family promoting good mental health.

The London Marathon is a behemoth, but it's hardly the only event out there. All over the country, and indeed the world, there are thousands of people, all lined up to push through aching knees and tired feet, to honour lost loved ones, bring awareness to mental health or collect money for a local community project. The people who run these kinds of races knock me out with their determination and good intentions. Many of them will have faced their own mental-health problems, or heartache, or tragedy. And yet they use their feet to do something for others. It's not just the personal challenge driving them on, it's a desire to use their sadness to stop others experiencing something similar. Next time you get an email asking for a donation, consider it. Few among us will put ourselves through such a challenge.

A close friend of mine died a few years ago, back in August 2015. Those around her felt the loss beyond words. This lively, hysterical, positive girl, who could leave us before she had even begun to show the world her full greatness. She was gone. But her sister, in the midst of her immense grief, signed up to run the London Marathon. She raised £26,000 which went to help those who were dealing with the illness that took her sister far too early. That kind of strength and determination is just hard to imagine when grief is threatening to envelop you. And yet she's doing it again. To remember her sister, to raise money, to stop it affecting another family. Running has become something else for the amazing people who run to honour lost loved ones, something to channel their energy into. Something which can sow positive seeds.

Michael and Rachel's son was stillborn. 'Ninety-nine per

cent of people would stop and ask how Rachel was,' Michael told me. 'No one would ask if I was OK. I would be told how I had to be strong for her. And so my mental health became affected. I smiled on the outside and broke on the inner. Simple tasks became a chore and I found myself wanting to hide away so I could cry in secret. Almost ashamed.'

Michael's experience with such tragedy is sadly not uncommon. The stillbirth and miscarriage charity Sands has said that more needs to be done to help men who are affected by stillbirth, as the focus is mainly on helping the mother through the experience.[106] Michael needed a focus for his grief, and he found it.

'I was always generally fit from my RAF days and I was asked to take part in a relay race three years after we lost Kyle. It gave me a taste of something new. I found I could put my music on and take my frustration out via my feet. It gave me an outlet I had never had before. And for my marathons, the feeling of pushing myself while raising money and awareness gave me a sense of belief. It was my therapy when I needed it most. From four-mile training to twenty, they all gave me a bubble away from reality.'

That might have been enough for most people. It helped him 'forget the world'. But Michael chose to do more with his running. 'My running has always been to honour Kyle. I feel that it's something he would want. My aim has always been to raise awareness of child loss, and fundraise in the hope that no other parent suffers as we did. If only one person sees our charity name or counts the kicks, it's potentially saving a life. We owe it to our son that he did not die in vain. Running is my therapy but also a great source of comfort for our whole family.'

Michael now runs to raise money for Sands, to help others

who have experienced such a loss, and to aid research which aims to prevent other families suffering the same. He has run six marathons and raised over £8,000 – he has a blog and you can find it at https://kylesdaddy.wordpress.com/. Please do go and read about his amazing work.

Obviously those who run to help others can also get something out of it for themselves – it would be a much harder, and perhaps less effective, challenge if running didn't also provide some comfort, or help build up some mental reserve. Michael sums up how it has helped him push forward, despite sadness, despite hurdles, despite life not going to plan:

'Running works perfectly for me. When we lost Kyle I was helpless. The same when cancer attacked my wife aged only twenty-six, and when my daughter was diagnosed with psoriasis aged five. Running is the one thing that I can control. I can push myself to limits I never knew I had. I can self-medicate and relieve any stress or tension finding my own peace in the highland air. Running gave me my confidence back. I can now write blogs and speak out. Before I could not. I guess I could say that running saved my life.'

It's not just individuals who use running to help other people. While I was writing this book, I got an email from a woman who wanted to tell me about the charity she ran with her partner. Wary of PR folks who try and shoehorn their products and campaigns into any communication, I was sceptical as to how relevant I would find their mission. But I read a bit about what they did, and my interest was pricked, so I duly went along and met the founder, Alex Eagle, at a local cafe. Over coffee, Alex explained that he'd worked at a homeless day centre for ten years, but was looking for something new and started up The Running Charity.

Believing that running builds resilience and boosts self-esteem, the charity offers exercise classes and running pro-grammes to 16–25-year-olds who are homeless or at risk of it. 'We partner with day centres and hostels, so we go to a place where they will be housed. We offer three fitness sessions per week there . . . We begin with a lot of stuff indoors and do personalised goal-setting plans with each young person – that can be as simple as getting them to turn up on time to them getting a job. There's lots of good charities out there for jobs, for housing. We're trying to improve people's mental health. That's what we're about.'

Alex started his charity from scratch, finding funding where he could, and working out of a shed to save money. But his belief in what running could do for vulnerable people held firm. And the stories he told back that belief up. After a young guy who'd been addicted to heroin completed his first Mud Run, he said to Alex: 'When I held that medal I knew I could achieve anything in my life.'

'And yeah that's it – that's the importance of the work. He took ownership of it,' Alex told me, looking proud. He believes that so often, the young people he works with have very little control over their lives. 'When a young person or anyone becomes homeless or goes through a difficult situation – when they put effort into fixing something it might not be fixed, because you go to a homeless shelter and there aren't any beds. You go to a job centre and you're sanctioned if you're a minute late. The odds are stacked against you.

'One of the beautiful things about running – or any type of fitness – is, if you do it for an hour, you'll probably be better the next time you do it. And there's a shift – actually I am in control of things, there's some basic element of your life that you do have control over. That's important for our young people. That can be the beginnings of something a lot better.'

With its humane and relaxed approach, plus its dedicated mentorship, The Running Charity has helped many young people living in difficult circumstances to find running and join a community. Alex emphasised the dangers of isolation and the growing number of people who come to the charity who've experienced it.

After Zamzam became a refugee, she was housed in a home for homeless young people whose staff teamed her up with the charity. They worked with Zamzam, who was one of two athletes representing her native Somalia at London 2012, competing in the Women's 400m. She now lives in private accommodation and continues to receive mentorship from Alex's team.

The passion that those involved have for what running can do, if I'm honest, might even beat mine. After a young mentee called Claude ran the marathon for the charity, a man from Manchester got in touch and wanted to get involved. 'We had no money but we gave him support and help to avoid pitfalls.' The man, whose name is George, quit his job of thirty years, re-mortgaged his house and he's now working full-time on the project. These people give up their free time, their energy and their experience, all because they know that running can change lives in ways much bigger and more lasting than many would believe.

'We're not trying to make marathon runners,' says Alex (though they have created more than a few). 'Running is a really powerful tool – even if you just do a park run every week you will feel better about yourself.'

# 8K - KNOW YOUR LIMITS

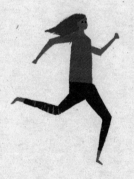

I ran around Oxford today. It's a brilliant place to run – the sheer amount of beautiful design in the city means you're constantly looking up, and stopping to gaze at ancient spires, stained glass, old pubs and worried-looking students. I could never finish university – anxiety took over that period of my life – so I'm still a little jealous of those who manage to enjoy a full scholarly experience. Aside from the cobbled streets and getting lost constantly, it's a great 8k, and I slow down to explore a bit more. As I'm turning onto the main shopping street, I encounter a horde of tourists complete with cameras, selfie sticks and backpacks. A stray foot connects with mine and I can feel the dreaded fall coming. I fall over *a lot* while I'm running. Maybe I'm clumsier than others, maybe my toes don't go the right way. Whatever it is, it's not unusual for me to stack it while I'm out and about. Knowing it's coming is the worst feeling. Every part of your body is panicking, trying to hold onto the air, flailing. And it never works. You have to just accept it and connect with the ground below. So I do. And I end up skidding along on my left thigh for a few seconds, ripping my leggings and leaving me in hiccupy tears as concerned tourists gaze down on me. Someone offers me a hand up, and I retrieve my smashed-up phone (I've broken this same phone eight times this way). I could shamelessly tell you that part of life is falling down and learning to get up, but I'm better than that. Or maybe I'm not. There is something hilarious about hopelessly tumbling in public, and there's something that makes you feel like a badass if you can get back up and run on. Or in this case, let the embarrassment fade and hobble off to get a chocolate bar to cheer myself up. I've still got a small scar on my hip from that run.

Why run a marathon?

I have told you that I am a bad runner. Maybe not *really* bad, maybe just a bit crap. I'm not being humble – I can put in the time, and I run most days. I psyched myself up to read the slightly intimidating book (one of our greatest living authors writes a brilliant running book: good subject for me to attempt, then) by the novelist Haruki Murakami, *What I Talk About When I Talk About Running*, and joyfully realised I was clocking up almost as many miles as him a week.[107] Only I've never got much faster than I did running up the alleyway, and I've never run much further than about 15k. I've never checked out my personal best and I've never even done as much as a half marathon, much less a full one. The idea fills me with dread, all those cheery people, some in ridiculous costumes, running for hours and then being wrapped in tinfoil blankets. And I haven't even included the weeks and months of training, eating well, going to sleep early and not drinking. *Noooooo* thank you.

So sometimes I feel like a fraud when I tell people I'm writing a book about running and they naturally assume I'm a hardened long-distance runner and proceed to ask me about my toughest experience. I don't usually tell them that the hardest run I've ever done took me just nine miles from my house and that I got so hungry I had to stop for a sandwich halfway through. But then, I was always intimidated by those brilliant marathon runners, and it never fuelled me to do it myself. It looked too hard, too joyless, too professional. So I tell you that I'm a bit rubbish at it, and hope you'll still listen to me when I argue that it's just as effective for you. Bryony Gordon also sees herself as a bad runner, and she's done the London Marathon, so I'm obviously not the only one.

That's not to say that you can't approach a marathon with a joyful and slightly amateurish mindset. In *Running Like a Girl* Alexandra Heminsley writes with such frankness and sheer optimism about doing a marathon (and then another, and another) that I almost wanted to sign up for a big race. Almost, mind. She writes that 'Every single training run suddenly made sense as my legs found the power to overtake handfuls of people . . . I wasn't a failure, I wasn't pathetic, I wasn't weak. I had proved that I could set a goal and meet it. I had shown that I could redefine who I was and who I could be.'[108]

There's something appealing about having a goal in mind, especially when you're depressed or anxious. The structure, the ambition not to let anyone down, and the pleasure of seeing yourself get better at something – I understand it all. But I'm now fiercely protective of my running time. I started it to get out of heartbreak and to stem the tide of anxiety. I wouldn't have imagined that it would end up bringing me joy and confidence and imbue me with a love of exercise, but here we are. And now I don't want to change something that isn't broken. I've discovered that there's no right way to run. There is an elderly man who lives near me and runs to the supermarket every day. He wears indecently short shorts and a sweatband like something out of a bad eighties movie, and it obviously works for him because he's remarkably speedy. I see a girl doing weird loops of a square nearby, and wonder why she doesn't extend her route until I remember that I couldn't leave an alleyway for weeks when I first started. Then there are the treadmill crew, who pound away in airless gyms and look grim-faced and angry. But they keep on keeping on, and they're not getting lost down side streets, sodden and windswept.

And then there are people who want to run for miles and miles. They want to run marathons, and then ultra-marathons. Ultra-marathons – anything longer than the normal twenty-six miles. One such runner, Zach Miller, often runs over a hundred miles. He described the feeling in an interview with the *Guardian*. 'Running is the closest we can get to flying . . . someone else said that, but I like it. For a brief moment, you're off the ground. And when you run as far as I do, you get lots of moments like that.'[109]

Sometimes the pain that these tough goals will bring is a tangible yardstick for how well you're doing. As Murakami writes in *What I Talk About when I Talk About Running*, 'It's precisely because of the pain, precisely because we want to overcome that pain that we get the feeling . . . of being really alive . . . or at least a partial sense of it.'[110]

For Nicola, who I talked about in my second chapter, her struggle with PTSD led her to running. 'I left the RAF in 2013, watched the London Marathon in 2015 and decided I would like to do it and take part, so I entered the ballot for it and started to train. I found that when I started to run it helped me to relax and be more happy in myself, and the more I did the better I felt. I managed to move to my own home and found a decent job – everything seemed to clicked into place.

'I got a place with the Invictus Games Foundation for April 2018. Since 2015, I have done over 95 races – anything from a mile to a hundred kilometres, the London to Brighton walk. Apart from running to help my PTSD, collecting medals seems to have become an obsession.'

Nicola finds that the challenges that races bring help with her mood. 'I am now much better in my mind. I do have the odd days when I feel everything is going against me, but the good days outweigh them now. I have my own flat in London and can now do what I like when I like. I have also started theatre work and become an extra for films and TV.'

All of these people have something in common. They are all runners. I have never wanted to push my body to run a hundred miles. I think I'd hate every minute of it, and lose the love of the pursuit. But I completely understand the strange and alluring feeling of 'flying' and I think all runners would say the same. One of the joys of trying it out for yourself is not knowing where it will lead you. My journey is probably one of medium-length runs and continuing to do it almost every day. Somebody else might do 5k twice a week and another person might get completely competitive and sign up for every race under the sun. I do it for my mind, others for their fitness, but we all reap the same benefits in the end.

My perfect run will be different from yours. It's usually a morning one – when I'm fully awake and usually feeling a little overwhelmed at what the day will bring – a deadline, bills that needs paying, little niggles which I can easily get fixated on. The first ten minutes hurt, without fail. I have to push myself to get that first ten done, and I always feel lumbering and slow initially, like the Tin Man clanking down the yellow brick road. After ten minutes, my body feels looser, and I'll finally stop focusing all my attention on willing it to carry on. From here on in, the good thing happens. My brain sort of 'detaches' from my body. I can feel my feet hitting the pavement, and I know I'm using my arms to pump. I'm there in the moment but also I'm not. My mind gets to drift slightly. Sometimes I just gaze at the buildings around me, or the greenery if I'm out of the city. Sometimes I remember times in the past which heave into view completely unprompted. Often, I'll think about bigger-picture stuff – my career, my loved ones, whether I want babies one day (though I've never answered this successfully on a run), but without panicking or tying my mind up in knots.

Thoughts come and go as I run, but nothing sticks, and nothing becomes intimidating or irrational. Usually a good run will take me past something I haven't seen before, or allow me the space to think about something differently, but if not, I don't worry. Occasionally a good run means thinking about nothing very much, but feeling comfortable about it. How often do we just allow our brains to zone out without feeling unproductive or searching for our phones or the laptop to plug ourselves back into the world? It often feels as though disconnecting for a bit is a cop-out – especially in an age when news is relentless.

I spent much of 2016 to 2017 working as a news editor. This was a marked change of pace after working on comment and opinion, which is frantic, but less so than news. Journalists often joked that 2016 could not be beaten for world events, and every hack I knew was exhausted going into the new year. That year was an anomaly, we were sure. EXCEPT WE WERE ALL WRONG – 2017 was a shitshow. The constant jaw-dropping moments began to roll into one – events that would have dominated the news cycle for days or even weeks flickered for mere hours before being overtaken by others that demanded attention too. Things that were shocking, tragic and just baffling were no longer necessarily affecting people as deeply as before – the constant merry-go-round of news wore people down and made them numb to it all. I remember being scared to go to the toilet on occasion, worried that I'd miss something major (this happened to both me and other colleagues in 2016 several times and we got paranoid). I once reported on a terrorist attack while sitting in a bar while everyone else got drunk. I spent a weird morning in a B&Q with my dad, who bought DIY stuff as I sat on some piles of laminate flooring trying to find a reporter to write about Fidel Castro dying.

The news was an onslaught and we were all able to read about what was happening in real time – via social media, flash alerts on our phone, live blogs, etc. The argument as to how much news you should consume is an ongoing one – some saying that it spikes anxiety by triggering cortisol levels and that what we consume can make us depressed and blunted, because, let's be honest, the news is normally of a negative slant.

But that was my job, so I consumed it all. From the moment I woke up, to the moment I went to bed. And in some bleak instances, even during the night – the shock Brexit result, delivered when most people had gone to bed assuming one outcome, meant I took no chances with the American election. Much good it did me. Or the world.

But the cycle pumped me full of stress hormones – my stomach felt full of twirling ballerinas kicking my insides and I started having tension headaches – a thing I'd not experienced since my early twenties when I thought I had a brain tumour. I'd dread waking up, knowing that something would've happened overnight that I'd be behind on, something to hastily scramble to cover. I woke up with anxiety coursing through me when I was twenty-two and I'd found myself in the same place when I was thirty-two. The anxiety was about a job, and not free floating, but it was there nonetheless.

But, BUT! I wasn't twenty-two. Thank fuck. I was a decade older, and somewhat wiser and I had tools. The main one being I could run it off. And this is when I found my favourite running sweet spot. This is when I put it to use. No more whimsical runs along canals; and across the city to sightsee; or to acclimatise myself with crowds; or even to knock off a hangover. This was a time when I needed to run off adrenaline, to have some time away from the computer, and to be unavailable. I decided to run home from work every day. I would ignore all messages while I was running and I'd only listen to music or podcasts which didn't mention any breaking news at all. I never wanted to do it. I'd change into my running clothes at the end of the day, when I was knackered and hungry and everyone else was going to the pub. I'd strap on my heaving backpack and endure the comments about how ridiculous I was, and get going. The route was always the same, which I struggle with – I normally want to find and see new things when I run – and it took thirty-eight minutes, much of it uphill. For me, as a pretty slow runner, that was just over six kilometres and every minute was usually a struggle. But I stuck to it, and ran home every day I worked in news, knowing that, for me, it was the most helpful thing I could do to relieve the pressure I felt from the onslaught of news. Once I was home, the weight had shifted, and my mind, calmed from the interlude, would be able to wind down slightly. I will always have a huge affection for the commuters who run, grim-faced, with their work clothes stuffed up in their backpacks, dodging through crowds and hurtling towards the calm of their couches. Even if they don't feel it at the time, they're giving themselves a vital break from daily life.

And that's the thing about finding something that helps with mental-health problems. I learnt I couldn't just run when I was heartbroken. I couldn't just run when I was trying to face down panic attacks. I had to do it even when I felt happy; or fine; or mildly stressed; or just tired. It wasn't a tool I could use only on the sunny days, or when I felt 'cured'. It was precisely the times when things were difficult but manageable that I had to do it. That I *still* have to do it. These are the times when things can slip without you realising – when old symptoms of anxiety can creep back in faster than you might imagine they could. Vigilance is key. That might sound like I'm advocating being hyper-aware at all times, but what I really mean is that you should check in on your emotions from time to time and not hope that you're all fixed and could never be blindsided by mental-health problems again.

I felt panicked by work, and slightly despairing at the deluge of horrifying news I had to cover. I know that my job was perhaps a niche example. But I also know everyone has times in their careers where things feel overwhelming and ultra-hard. And my decision to run home every day is something that, as I did it, I saw mimicked by so many others. Men and women across the city, with their heavy backpacks and grim expressions of determination. Those who shrugged off the anxieties of work by pounding home, rather than sitting on the train and dwelling on the day.

And that's how I found my sweet-spot run. I'd always been pushing myself to run faster and longer, thinking that I could only be a 'proper' runner if I did a race, or committed to a training routine, or joined a running club. I never did any of these things, but I would still berate myself for only running 10k, doing it slowly, or doing it alone. The runs I did every weekday for a year while I was working in a stress-filled job were not my ideal runs. They were carthorse runs, no elegant stallions to be seen. But they were a tonic on days when I found my brain whirring. They were functional runs, all done to get home as quickly as possible; through dark streets, in the rain, and even in the snow on occasion. No runner's high. No bouncy elation from racing downhill. But I'd get home, and feel like I'd shrugged off the adrenaline of the day. I'd be able to answer emails, or keep track of the news again, knowing I'd taken thirty-eight minutes out of my day to just shut my brain off and move. It meant when I woke up the next morning, I'd feel the adrenaline kick off and know that I could shut it down later on in the day. At twenty-two, I had been in the grip of this every day. Now I could, if not rid myself of it entirely, control it, hem it in.

Thirty-eight minutes a day. Not a marathon. Not a half-marathon. Not even a 10k. But a check on my mental-health woes, which had held me prisoner for so many years. That's what worked for me. Any more and I was exhausted; any less and my brain wouldn't switch off. When I left that job, I rediscovered longer and more joyful runs and I experimented with early-morning sprints. But that period of my life taught me that running was something I'd signed up to for the long term. It didn't always have to be fun. It didn't even need to be long. It served me in a new and regimented way. I had to fit it in around something bigger – as most people do. It wasn't a luxury that I could revel in; it was a vital part of my day which helped me do everything else. Like I say, you find your own sweet spot, and the magic of running is that it can change from day to day. Someone else might be able to do their job magnificently without any crutch. Some people could do it with a weekly run, or a yoga session or a delicious dinner. But I needed that specific time out, and nothing else would have given it to me. Well, that and wine. Wine always makes a huge difference for me. But unlike running, this is not advised by your doctor. Sadly.

Runners can be pretty evangelical, I don't know if that's come through here at all (for the benefit of the tape, this is a joke). Everyone who runs (OK, maybe not everyone, but I've yet to find someone who defies this rule) lights up when someone else mentions they do it too. It's like the opposite of a secret society. But invariably, that eagerness to share the joy of it means telling people how they should do it. 'Oh you haven't done hill sprints up Ben Nevis? You must, it's a different level. I do it every morning. Before my commute to Brighton.' That's a fairly smug example, actually: I'm being unfair. And I just made it up, too. So let's strike that from the record. After all, I've written a whole book about why you should run. But I've been intimidated many a time by runners who have pushed themselves further than I ever will. It's all well meaning, but sometimes it can shake your own expectations of running. Far better to start small and find your own sweet spot. That being said, LET ME NOW DISPENSE MORE

ADVICE – I promise none of it involves hill sprints or back-wards running (which someone did once urge me to try).

I've said before that I'd recommend the Couch to 5K programme to anyone seeking to start running from the scary position of never having done it even once. That's where I really got hooked. The clear progress I was making buoyed me, and made me keep going back. (As an aside, do apps which remind you constantly that you're failing to keep up with their programmes give anyone else an existential crisis?) But it's not the only way to kick off your running . . . I don't ever want to use the word journey . . . arghh . . . umm . . . *experiment*. Phew. Running clubs are hugely popular – google England Athletics to find a local one near you. I've said I prefer to run alone, but, despite this, I've found time goes much faster when you're with a pal. And the encouragement of others might really help you keep at it. If I hadn't been so ill and irrational and negative when I started, I might well have been more open to joining a club myself. For those who have built up some initial runs, Parkrun is a great initiative – based on their original principle of 'weekly, free, 5km, for everyone, forever'. There are 497 different locations in the UK and they've expanded to other countries too – so if you're abroad and wanting to run but don't know where, their website has a handy map of all of their locations. You can go at your own pace, and the atmosphere is welcoming and warm.

Gyms are stuffed with running machines, if you don't fancy braving the cold weather – which is basically nine months of the year. The instructors are usually happy to help you discover all the features on the treadmills – you can opt for different programmes and some fancy ones even have TV channels or (my favourite) the option to run virtually –

following a video of a trail somewhere else in the world. I had a friend who only ran LA beaches for six months as she was getting over a break-up. Every time I saw her on the treadmill she'd be watching a screen which showed sun and crashing waves and buffed bodies strolling beside her. It was quite the juxtaposition to the grey London days outside. I've never much got on with running machines. Not being able to vary my pace naturally frustrates me, and I like to be outside. But they're efficient and get you moving, and sometimes when I'm travelling, all I want is to get a run out of the way – and a treadmill is perfect for this. If you get on with it, then great, but I'd always recommend going outside and trying to run there too – even just to make sure you're not missing out. I'm sceptical that you can get all the mental-health benefits if you're not getting the vitamin D and the added benefit of people-watching and (if you're lucky) seeing some greenery.

However you do it, set reasonable expectations for yourself – and decide what you want to get out of it. I stuck at it, having previously dropped anything I found hard, because I started so small. One minute at a time. Yes it hurts, yes your muscles will ache tomorrow. But you can do one minute. Don't rashly decide to run for thirty minutes when you're feeling sad or anxious – if you can't manage it, you'll feel like you've failed at something, and that's a terrible feeling even if you're not already having a hard time. Try to mix running with walking – when it feels too hard, just slow down until you feel ready to go again. If you feel like you might be having a panic attack, focus on your breathing – running can make you out of breath and you might misconstrue that as panic. I did this a few times at the beginning – it's funny to learn that the physical symptoms of anxiety can be mimicked by intense cardio exercise – racing heart, sweat, flushed face, pounding head. You just have to slow down and work out whether these things dissipate when you're not working your body so hard. Ninety-five per cent of the time my body was just reacting normally to doing something strenuous for the first time in years.

Remember that you might not feel any immediate difference – I felt something change on my first run, but that was probably only because a curiosity had been sparked in me, rather than that I had hit some physical high (I had definitely not earned one). When I drag myself out of bed to go for a run now, I remind myself that I never feel *worse* afterwards. Maybe you might keep this mantra too – you might not feel like all your anxieties have left you initially, but you won't feel worse. Well, maybe a bit knackered.

Bethany remembered what running could offer when she was hit with a deluge of problems. Her relationship wasn't going well, her job was difficult and she was going through an incredibly difficult court case. She'd run when she was younger, she told me, before anxiety and depression had hit her aged eighteen. She'd stopped as an adult – work and family coming first. But when she found herself unable to get out of bed in April 2017, she knew that her mental-health problems had returned with a vengeance.

'I have a young son and he doesn't deserve to see me like this. He didn't deserve to watch his mum cry in a ball every single day. It took me a while to figure out what I needed to do, then I remembered how running made me feel. Remembering that feeling made me determined to go outside and run, for as long and as far as I possibly could. I wasn't training for anything, this was purely to remind myself how free I can feel just by running.'

Bethany didn't set herself any running goals at all. She just went out and did it, hoping it would make a difference, suspecting that, as it had before: 'My mind would clear and I'd forget all my worries.' I think this is really intuitive exercise; Bethany ran for as long as she felt she needed to feel better. No expectations, no setting herself up for failure. She already felt like she was doing everything in her life badly, but with this: 'It wasn't something I could do "wrong", which was my mentality at the time. I felt I couldn't do a single thing right, but with running it didn't matter. I could just go and nothing was holding me back.'

Since she started running again, Bethany has found her depression and anxiety loosening their grip. 'I dip in and out of low patches. I'm a lot better than I was and I credit a lot of that to running. It's a way to get out of my own head.'

By taking things easy, Bethany didn't expect too much, or berate herself when she didn't feel better within days. She has slowly begun to feel better, and picked up a habit at the same time.

Alexandra Heminsley met Paula Radcliffe (three-time winner of the London Marathon, amazing woman with legs of steel) while writing her book about running.[111] She asked her what her advice would be for someone thinking about trying it out. 'Just . . . go out and try it. Do it. Go out and have fun, see if you like it,' said Radcliffe. It might not be the most original wisdom ever imparted, but it's accurate. Try it out. See what happens. And if you're feeling trapped in your brain, and desperate to get out, running just might be the way out. At the beginning, my brain would give me reasons not to go out and run. And I would have to argue back. Eventually I just started blocking the thoughts by speaking out loud.

'Why not?' I'd ask the empty room. 'What have you really go to lose?' And I'd go.

So if your brain is resisting like mine was – go ahead and ask the question – what have you really got to lose? Your brain might find some pretty miserable answers, but they're all likely to be straw men. And the more you do it, the more you knock those straw men down.

# 9k – LISTENING TO YOUR BODY

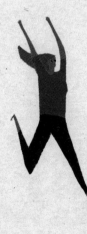

I'm running up a hill with my ex-boyfriend. We broke up when I was twenty-one, but we've kept in touch sporadically. Nobody broke anyone's heart, we were just young and we (me in particular) had no idea how to have a relationship. Marios has embarked on a mission that seems ludicrous — he's going to run through jungle in South America (where is never really stipulated), doing six marathons in six days for charity. At high altitude. He's not really much of a runner, but a career in mixed martial arts means he's fit as anyone can be. I don't think he loves to run, though, not really. So I offered to go with him, and now we're pounding up a hill, urging each other onwards. Back when we dated, I was a sad and overweight girl prone to spontaneous bouts of crying, who had a constant urge to eat family bags of crisps. He was a fitness fanatic who weighed his meals and took the skin off chicken because it was needlessly fatty. We were a weird match. Now our physicality has almost met in the middle, and I have no problem pacing him. I'm entranced by how much he's making me laugh, despite the cold and the stitch I get halfway in. We race over Hampstead Heath, and push on down through Swiss Cottage and onto the Finchley Road, passing our old haunts and talking about all the stupid fights we used to have. It's a run through memories, those which make us laugh but also which make me feel strangely detached from my past. It's odd to remember being so deeply lost and unhappy, as though it was all happening to someone else. I feel like a completely different person, someone who found an even keel by luck. Marios is kind about the past, even though I must've been a nightmare to date. It's hard to go out with someone who doesn't know anything about who they are.

We carry on through, down to Regent's Park, stopping to have a go on the see-saw in the children's playground, and to twirl around on the tiny swings. I take a photo of us giggling on the roundabout, before I make him complete the loop and run me home. We finish feeling bouncy and childish – more proof to me that every run I complete prompts a completely different reaction, and can throw up unexpected realisations. I feel like I've come a long way, something I'd not seen so clearly since I started running. Marios never completed his big trip, by the way; an injury forced his early retirement from the race, and he hasn't asked me to run since.

We know that most people do not do the suggested amount of exercise recommended by the NHS – indeed in 2017, Public Health England (PHE) said that 41 per cent of English adults aged 40 to 60 walk less than 10 minutes continuously each month at a pace of at least 3 mph.[112] On top of that, the same report showed that a quarter of the English population do less than thirty minutes of exercise a week – classing them as 'inactive'.

I find it easy to understand this, having spent much of my life mostly sedentary. But because running has enriched my mind and mood as well as my physical body, I also know how exercise has now woven itself into my day, into my being, without me making a conscious decision to allow it to. I can't go a day without doing it, for so many reasons. To wake me up properly; to stop my mind whirring; to stave off anxiety and depression in the future; and to allow my brain space to switch off. And from doing it, I have come to realise how often we separate our minds and our bodies – how we value our intelligence, our learning and our thinking over our feet, our knees, our backs. In other words, we see our very being as split between the mental and the physical. But this is so misguided. 'A sick thought can devour the body's flesh more than fever or consumption.' Guy de Maupassant was bang on.

In Damon Young's book *How to Think About Exercise*, he begins by saying that so many people see a conflict between mental and physical exertion – and value one but not the other. 'We grow accustomed to a professional life in which labour – and often identity – is chiefly mental not physical, and interaction virtual. We still have bodies of course, but their contribution to character is diminished.'[113]

Our lifestyles mean that we often let our bodies come second to everything else. Too tired, too busy, hate the gym, would rather see friends. As Haruki Murakami says in *What I Talk About When I Talk About Running*, 'If I used being busy as an excuse not to run, I'd never run again.'[114] And I understand that. Lives are full and exercise seems like something either too worthy or merely vapid and self-indulgent. A low priority, in other words. But seeing it in these terms, we further disconnect our minds from our bodies. If we view exercise as hard, or narcissistic, we make it easier to avoid doing altogether.

Have you ever heard of a Blue Zone? It's a term coined to explain the places where the world's oldest people reside. In 2005 Dan Buettner identified nine places where those ancient people live – and explained what factors kept them going for so long.[115] One of those factors was . . . yeah, obviously, it was exercise. But not just any old exercise – not twenty minutes on a rowing machine and then going back to your desk for the rest of the day. The exercise was threaded throughout life – shepherds in Sardinia, for example, who walked for miles each and every day. There were other factors that led to their longevity, like minimal alcohol intake and regular social interaction, but the importance of activity has always stuck with me.

As Buettner said in a 2015 interview: 'Our team found that people [in these places] are nudged into physical activity every twenty minutes or so . . . They're walking to their friend's house. They're going down to the garden. They're kneading bread with their hands. It's natural movement. It's something they don't have to think about. It's not something that requires discipline.'

The way these older people incorporated exercise was not to see it as exercise at all, but part of life – not a punishment or a chore, but something like lunch, happening regularly, and never with a definite start and stop.

Vybarr Cregan-Reid told me that while we now see ourselves as physically fit if we do thirty minutes in the gym a couple of times a week, we might be deluding ourselves somewhat. [116]

'Today, we think of people as being active or sedentary. Lots of people now think as long as you exercise regularly, you're fine. But then if you spend the rest of your time being sedentary, you're not shielding yourself from diseases like diabetes. It's not enough.'

Vybarr also praised the lifestyle of the Sardinian shepherds: 'They walk anywhere from five to nine miles a day, which is the same as hunter-gatherers used to do. They're burning calories at a higher level than someone who's sedentary.'

This approach is rare in the modern world. I don't do it as effortlessly as the Sardinians. But the more I ran, the more I wanted to move my entire body. And not so I could see visible muscles; or make my arse look better in jeans; but because I finally understood how my mind and my body are working in tandem all the time. For most of my life I have been trapped by my mind, afraid and tense. I used to get incredible head-aches – the kind which floor you with pain, hovering over your eyes and making movement a risky business when you know nausea is right around the corner. I never connected them with anxiety, I just took loads of paracetamol and tried to get on with stuff. I would willingly believe that my physical symptoms were the early signs of something chronic and terrifying, but would dismiss any mental connection as hocus pocus. I resided in my body, but I kept it still, hunched and humming with adrenaline.

I didn't give my mind enough credit for the sheer fucking determination and will it had. It could make me feel like I had the flu; hunch me over with backache; give me headaches; make me so cold I'd always wear puffer jackets in the office in July. All anxiety – why was that so hard to accept? It was because I was separating my mind from my body, imagining they worked in offices in different cities and never communicated. I was an idiot.

It still amazes me how long I spent living not just with mental discomfort, but with physical ailments too. I felt run down and exhausted nearly all the time. I would get woozy with fatigue during the day, and then face sleepless nights because every part of my body would be freezing, shivering under four blankets. I was so concerned with my mind that I just assumed my body would always feel like this and did my best to ignore it all. Running did what doctors never could – though my GP tried many times. It made me understand how closely the two are linked. If I felt like a load was lifted during the early jogs I took – less crying, fewer panic attacks – that was nothing compared to realising that every run I took not only made my mind feel better, but also diminished the physical ailments that I assumed I was stuck with. Yes, I got more flexible, and slept better, but my headaches didn't suddenly disappear purely from physical exertion. They faded, gradually, until one day I couldn't remember the last time I'd had one. This coincided with a lessening of adrenaline churning in my stomach, and a cessation in my almost constant teeth-grinding (yes I should have worn a retainer to bed, but I couldn't face the ignominy). I slowly understood that the main thing that connected all of these things was simple: I was happier.

Once I figured this out, I began to try and listen to my body more. If I felt uptight, coiled like a spring when I woke up, that meant I was feeling worried about something. From that, there were two options. Option one was to figure out what was bothering me, and option two was to go for a run. Sometimes I'd do both. Sometimes going for a run made me realise what was wrong, and sometimes it gave me the chance to put it in perspective.

When I felt tired, I would go for a walk, knowing that I needed to inject some fresh air (as fresh as Zone One in London can get) and not allow myself to sleepily carry on at half speed. This could be just ten minutes, but it always made a noticeable difference, and I do it all the time now. I walk in the mornings before I even have a cup of coffee. It gives me space between deep sleep and the busy day, time to fully let my brain wake up, so I don't jolt it into panic with a rush to the Tube or by expecting to start work straight away.

When I feel low, my instinct is normally to sweat through it – which usually means weights, squats and other slightly torturous exercises, which make me feel a bit stronger, as though my reserves aren't totally empty. This also works for hangovers, by the way.

But even when I'm not feeling any of those things, I try and keep on weaving the thread of physical movement throughout my life. I enjoy moving everything now. A stretch which wakes up a previously dormant muscle feels exciting. Legs which hurt the day after weights make me happy because I've woken up a bit of me which has been underused. I get up and down and feel restless at a desk in a way I never expected. The feeling of vegging on the sofa holds less appeal than it used to, which is a double-edged sword, to be honest. Motivation is key in all of this, and sometimes it's just as hard to get up and exercise when you're happy as it is when you're incredibly sad.

Falling in love again knocked me off course. Partly because it seemed like something which wouldn't happen, certainly not with the intensity and happiness that it did. As the relationship progressed, I dropped running every day and walking every morning for lie-ins and long dinners. Somehow it all felt too hard to do when there were such lovely options calling me. And for a while, I gave in to them. There were days where I didn't move my body at all. And they were very nice. I argued that I was just having a break from the daily slog, that I deserved to slack off for a bit. But that was a mistake, because I was starting to look at running in terms of punishment, and forgetting what it gives me. I didn't feel increasingly anxious or sad – the contrary, I was all soppy and glowing – but I knew that stopping the very thing that had given me the tools to have a good relationship would be a mistake. Running wasn't a means to an end; it was to aid the whole journey.

I'm sure you've heard the tired old cliché that you put on weight at the beginning of a new relationship. Well, it's certainly tired, but it's not untrue. After too many lingering dinners and croissants for breakfast, I realised I had fallen into the trap. And so I started running every day again. Not the most noble or worthy reason to return to it, I admit, but it got me back in the stride. I'd only slacked off for a couple of months, but I took the itch to get back into running regularly as a sign of the stronger connection I now had to my body. And I needed that unique feeling of being on my own with my thoughts after a period away from it. Being coupled up can mean much less time alone. And it's nice, but I'd only recently learnt to enjoy it, so I wasn't going to let that go.

When I started running, I often felt very lonely – I was adjusting to being on my own again, and found it very difficult to spend too much time without the company of others. In getting married and hunkering down, I'd neglected my social life and become too scared to go out much. While people rallied round, they obviously had their own lives to live, and I couldn't rely on others for everything. Even my sister, who had stayed for weeks, had to go back to her flat at some point.

If the feelings of isolation got too much, and I started to feel anxious because of them, I'd go running. The stress of feeling alone is well documented. According to government figures, young people – those between sixteen and twenty-four – are more likely to report feeling alone than previously.[117] The UK has even appointed a Minister for Loneliness to try and combat the rise of isolation, because certain research suggests that loneliness increases the likelihood of mortality by 26 per cent.

If I spend too long on my own, I notice my anxiety levels shooting up. I start noticing irrational thoughts creeping in, and I begin to feel jittery. I went through a period of feeling pretty alone when my marriage broke up – partly that's just to be expected when someone permanently vacates your life. But partly, I wasn't being particularly proactive. I didn't want to bother people more than I already had. And so I found myself spending some weekends never seeing another soul. And I wasn't about to encourage those anxious feelings I could feel creeping in, making themselves at home again, regaining what I'd reclaimed. So I would go running. Sometimes I'd run around the park and go home having had just enough of an interlude to feel OK about returning to an empty flat. But sometimes that wouldn't be enough, and I'd use the running time to take me somewhere – a cafe, or a museum, or just a trip to the shops. I often found myself discovering places I'd never seen or previously ignored. My eyes were open to my surroundings and I took immense joy in noticing a strange house, an old pub, a railway line hidden from normal view. I sometimes encountered the surreal – a group of rowdy Santas I had to weave through; a dog which took off from its owner and ran with me in the park; a man *swimming* down the London canal. Do you know how mucky that canal is? Not to mention the mardy swans. I love animals as much as the next weird person who pets strange dogs in the park, but swans are mean and rude. Don't fight me.

Dragging myself back from my irrational fury with swans, where was I? Yes, strangely, while I was going out on jogs, I never felt alone. I felt connected with my surroundings, woven into a tableau which included families out in the park, dog walkers, tourists and commuters. I'd pass fellow runners and push myself further, knowing I could do it if they could. Gwyneth Paltrow was laughed at a couple of years ago for promoting 'earthing' – which was described on her hilarious website Goop (go and have a look, if you need a blanket for your dog which costs 800 dollars). The language was fancy and lacking in plain English, but it basically boiled down to an argument that 'physically connecting to the planet is good for both the body and soul'. I think her version of earthing involved going barefoot on hand-fed grass or something equally bananas, but I felt something embarrassingly similar in those lonely moments. When I ran, I would feel connected with the world around me – part of something larger than just my neuroses. With every strike of my foot, I would calm down, feel less manic about the silence in my flat, realise that there was a world around me that I wanted to engage with and could, whenever I liked.

Being outside and moving for a while meant that I could go home and not feel separate, or 'other'. I could go home and do something vaguely productive rather than sit and silently get more and more agitated. So much of my life has been spent not feeling comfortable in my head, and loneliness only exacerbates this feeling – after all, loneliness can lead to mental-health problems. In 2014, researchers at the University of Chicago found that loneliness is a good predictor for future depressive symptoms.[118] But strangely, being alone while I was running felt good – it always feels good. Being on my own when I pound the pavements never seems weak, or pathetic – as it can do when you're rattling around an empty flat. It feels strong and deliberate. By linking my body to my brain better, and taking it out for a breather, I don't feel disconnected – I feel whole. *How to Think About Exercise* by Damon Young starts by talking about the mistake of 'dualism' – seeing your brain and body as separate entities. Because thinking 'does not happen away from the body'.[119] You can feel lonely in your mind, and still choose to be physically alone. And sometimes, as I found with running, you can merge the two things and end up OK.

Many people recommend running in nature to fully experience mind-boosting benefits. A 2015 Stanford University study set out to see if exercise in the outdoors would have any effect on the ruminations and worries associated with mental-health issues like depression.[120] The study had one group of participants take a 90-minute walk in a natural setting. The other group walked for the same duration and with the same intensity, but in an urban setting. The people who took their walk in nature reported decreased rumination, and scans of their brains also showed decreased neural activity in an area of the brain associated with mental illness (the subgenual prefrontal cortex). The group who walked in the city, however, experienced neither of these effects.

The study was small – just thirty-eight people – but I can see the argument. Walking in the countryside (a thing I have come to love now I'm older) always sets me up for the day in a way a city run can't quite manage. There's nothing like being alone and surrounded by beauty to calm jangled nerves. Especially with the magical silence the countryside offers. But that doesn't mean I derive nothing from a city jaunt. Many of us don't have a wide choice of fields and woodland in easy reach – recent UK government figures estimated that about 82 per cent of us live in urban areas.[121]

But for those who are lucky enough to have access to hills and moors and cliff tops, the experience can be profound. In *Running Free: a Runner's Journey*, journalist Richard Askwith describes how he initially started running in South London, and quickly fell in love with the sport.[122] He timed himself, and strove to run faster, longer, better – until it became thankless and too much like work. Askwith discovered running in nature, and changed his running outlook dramatically. He embraces rural running and revels in charging through rural Northamptonshire; in the changing seasons; in the animals and in the trips taken through muddy fields with his dog. Most interestingly, he rails against the commercialisation of running – the expensive kit, the obsession with personal bests, the corporate sponsorship of group runs, all of which he argues take away from the sheer joy of getting out and running for the sake of it. Vybarr Cregan-Reid also believes that it can be helpful to see running as 'not exercise'. 'Exercise is something that is mechanistic – you do it for a specific outcome . . . to get a healthy heart or to help with diabetes. Running is a lot more than a means to lose some weight. It's a multi-dimensional thing that's much much bigger than just exercise.'

Vybarr also put me onto the novel idea of 'forest bathing', when I asked how important nature is when doing physical activity.[123] It sounded slightly eccentric to my ignorant ears when he first raised it, but it tallies with the rise in environmental psychology research – a field which explores the relationship between people and their surroundings. Forest bathing is not having a bath in some woods – which I was initially excited about, if I'm honest.

Instead, researchers in Japan have studied what spending time in a forest can do for health problems such as high blood pressure. In 2010, the Centre for Environment, Health and Field Sciences at Chiba University studied the practice known as 'forest bathing,' or *shinrin-yoku*, in an attempt to measure the health effects on 280 people in their early twenties.[124] The researchers measured the pulse rate, salivary cortisol (which increases with stress), blood pressure and heart rate of those who spent half an hour in a forest during a day. These results were then compared with those taken during a day in the city. The outcome was pretty remarkable and the study ended by stating:

'Forest environments promote lower concentrations of cortisol, lower pulse rate, lower blood pressure, greater parasympathetic nerve activity, and lower sympathetic nerve activity than do city environments.'

Another Japanese study in 2007 used a larger group of subjects to research the benefits of forest bathing. Four hundred and ninety-eight healthy people spent a day in a forest, completing surveys twice in that time. 'Compared with the control day, the results showed that hostility and depression scores decreased significantly, and liveliness scores increased significantly on the forest day compared with the control day.'[125]

In addition, the study showed that 'stress levels were shown to be related to the magnitude of the *shinrin-yoku* effect; the higher the stress level, the greater the effect.'

This research revealed that forest environments can be helpful for those experiencing difficult emotions, especially those experiencing chronic stress. But forests are not the only environments that can help improve mood and lessen stress. Luckily for me, Vybarr reassured me that my running routes through parks and down canals will also help – anywhere with greenery, any place with a hint of nature. And if you look hard enough, you can find nature springs up in the most unlikely of places.

'Environmental psychology – anything where nature is involved always comes out better,' Vybarr told me. 'People coming out of hospital sooner because they have a view of greenery, a housing project in Chicago where the crime rate was lower in the areas where people who could see greenery lived.'

Cregan-Reid and Askwith are hardly alone in their passion for the outdoors and the benefits it can bring us. The mental-health charity Mind has long championed 'Ecotherapy' as one way to help tackle mental-health issues. Along with programmes encouraging people to spend more time in nature, their argument is bolstered by research by the University of Essex which showed that engaging in exercise while viewing images of beautiful green landscape improved self-esteem and lowered blood pressure. Further studies at the same university reported that 'green' exercise activities, like cycling, fishing and riding, made participants significantly less angry and depressed afterwards.

Mind identifies four key principles for ecotherapy.[126]

*Natural and social connections*
*Sensory stimulation*
*Activity*
*Escape*

Looking back at my lonely period, I recognise that these were the things I was unknowingly seeking when I went out to run. And I can also see that they were the things that helped me shrug off the worst of my anxiety, even though I didn't know it at the time. Mental-health issues can rob you of all of these human needs. For me, I missed out on real connection with both the world around me and the people I loved – never mind the people I was yet to meet. I avoided sensory stimulation, fearing it would kick off some new panic, and I certainly never tried any form of activity which might have propelled me out of my shell. I stayed small and confined. And that just leaves escape. Escape is a word I'm aware I've used a lot while writing this book. Escape from sadness, from anxiety, from my own brain. Not a permanent escape, but a brief moment of being 'away' from it all. It can be hard to put into words what an escape can bring you, but I can see how nature magnifies the effect, and makes the minutes you venture out of your comfort zone seem more meaningful, more worthwhile. As Carl Jung said, 'Whenever we touch nature we get clean.'[127]

Ever since I realised that running in nature could do more for my mind than city trails, I've been keen to try it whenever I travel. I once ran along the coast in Ireland, in a remote place that I'd never previously been before. I was fairly hungover, and just wanted to clear my head before I assumed bridesmaid duties, and had to give a speech and look presentable. In a

week in which a good friend had died, and another had had
a baby, I was already full up with emotions, and needed some
air and some time on my own. As I got further and further
away from the village, and nearer to the sea, I quickly realised
I was encountering the most beautiful scenery I'd ever seen.
Wind whipped around me, and gulls were the only companions
as I pushed forward. The light kept changing! The sky would
be blue and cool one minute, and then flip – brightening and
intensifying, until I was under bright sun. I ran past giant old
boats left out to wither, in the shadow of a mountain behind
me. I took in everything; even the air felt more tangible as it
buffeted me.

I'd left with swirling thoughts of death and life and babies
and here I was, ten minutes in, all of that forgotten. I only
saw the landscape, I *felt* my surroundings. The connection I
felt to the present was astounding to me – used to my city
life, and my busy brain – always focused on the past, on the
future, on 'what if' thoughts. Sakyong Mipham calls this
connection to our surroundings 'panoramic awareness'[128] and
it did feel like a sort of meditation, something I've never
thought I could do. I ran on easily, enjoying the steps, thinking
of nothing very much. I didn't feel sad or happy exactly, I just
felt very 'there'. And I was never smaller than on that run.
Smaller, but not diminished. I just had a flash of clarity, realising my connection to the world, and my tiny place in it.
Dr Mihaly Csikszentmihalyi termed this feeling 'flow' back
in 1975, though there are many other names for it, and he
described the factors it involves, which include:

• Complete concentration on the task
• A clear goal and immediate feedback

- The experience has an end, and is rewarding
- Effortlessness and ease
- A balance between challenge and skill
- Action and awareness are combined
- You feel in control of the task[129]

Sounds like a lot of work to get there, huh? Csikszentmihalyi says it takes work, for sure. You have to cultivate it. But that doesn't mean homework and mental dissection. For me, it just meant running regularly. And it's not just found in running, though for the purpose of this book, which is about running, it is. What I felt on that Irish expedition was most likely flow. It seemed different from the famous 'runner's high', though it shared similar characteristics. Not euphoria alone, but a general sense that I was right where I was supposed to be, doing what I should be doing. In effect, it was the opposite of my usual state. If anxiety is a feeling of panic, of doubt and of helplessness, that particular 'flowy' run felt calm; I had a certainty in what I was doing, and a sense of control. Perhaps it felt so extraordinary because, as an anxious person, I'm just not used to those sensations.

David, who suffers from generalised anxiety disorder (see this book's second chapter), told me that he finds a measure of flow in his runs too. 'The rhythmic, repetitive action of running gives me another focus – and doing a certain distance or breaking a certain time gives me an objective, measurable form of accomplishment which I don't get from many other things. It's the only "method" I have found which works for me in switching my focus away from intrusive thoughts. So I should get out there more often, really!'

I think I'll remember that run forever. Partly because I cried when I took a break midway to just watch the waves and hear the sea, so overwhelmed by the whole thing. I'll be grateful that I experienced such clarity and such a unique feeling of being in the moment (I know, what a clichéd phrase). But I don't seek it in every run, and to do so would be counterproductive, diluting every other run I do, which all have their rewards. I mention it only because running is the only activity which has rewarded me with 'flow', and given me such peace. And I'd never have imagined it was possible. And it encapsulates why I'm so passionate about such a simple activity (just in case I haven't conveyed it adequately enough already).

Although I've mostly concentrated on how running has dramatically reduced my anxiety and allowed me to untangle my thoughts, perhaps I haven't mentioned another important reason for this. In the midst of endorphins, or a serotonin boost or being in nature or finding a flow state, I forgot to mention self-esteem. Something that magazines go on about a lot – finding it, boosting it, keeping it. But I'd never connected it to me. I was negative about myself, and described myself in jokingly dismissive ways, but it never occurred to me that perhaps I didn't really have any confidence.

I quit things when they got hard, and I hid from stuff I was scared of (read: most things), and these traits meant I slowly just decided I couldn't really do much of anything. But in a funny way, I'd decided that was OK, as long as I always joked about it and never made a serious confession to anyone about not liking myself. I think a lot of people do what I did, especially women. I certainly wasn't uniquely crippled by a lack of confidence. Or so I thought. But then, I never applied for jobs, or struck out and tried new challenges. I let men treat me pretty shoddily. I was grateful for any praise, but would normally bat it off.

Getting a divorce will seriously affect any confidence or 'self-esteem' you might have cultivated. And if that's not enough, anxiety will deftly get rid of the rest. But it never has to be gone forever. And trying out a new hobby or learning a new skill can boost your sense of self surprisingly quickly. As with most things, duality is key. You might feel good about your mental abilities but hate how physically weak you feel. You might be able to do fifty push-ups in a row but feel useless in your career.

The trick is to work on both. Easier said than done, obviously. I started growing in confidence every time I ran a bit longer, or dragged myself out in the pouring rain, I felt like I was banking small achievements. I didn't give up after a week – one boost. I ran 5k in one go – another noticeable lift. Every time I laced up my trainers while secretly longing to stay indoors, I felt proud of myself.

The absolutely brilliant thing about starting a new habit for yourself (and not doing it as part of a team) is that you don't have anyone to fail. Of course, having others taking part too gives you extra accountability, but sometimes even that level of pressure might be too much. I wasn't ready for that. I just wanted to try something out, and place no expectations on it. Hence starting my running attempts in a dark alley. Nobody to watch, nobody to laugh, and nobody to judge me if I stopped.

You can't measure self-esteem, but there are some generally accepted signs that you have a healthy level of it. They include an ability to make mistakes and learn from them, optimism, assertiveness, being able to trust others, and good self-care.

Without confidence, it's easy to fall into depression, fear failure and avoid taking any risks. Tick, tick, tick!

Charities such as Mind suggest you try a new hobby or learn a new skill if you're looking to grow your confidence. So I was doing something right, even if I didn't know it. The first time I ran for a kilometre without stopping, I skipped home. Literally. I was so pumped to have that distance under my belt that I was bouncy enough not to care what I looked like as I went. And I didn't need to tell anyone to make it better. I had it in my brain, and that was enough.

Confidence breeds confidence, or maybe it just lessens the fear of failure. While my anxiety receding was the main joy I took from running, I did notice that I also felt so much better about myself as a person. Those niggling doubts over things I'd said or done during the day, which used to keep me up for hours, would give up within minutes. I'd feel like I could speak up in meetings, or ask for a pay rise. Without a boost in confidence, none of this would've been possible. I even felt able to confront the fears – now I had some gas in the tank – that I'd avoided forever. And even some that I didn't know I had . . .

It was 3pm and sunny as I strolled through Regent's Park in London. Children ran about, frisbees were thrown. Ice creams were being licked all around me. So why did I think I was about to lose control of all my bodily functions?

The answer loomed large in front of me. Through the trees, just past the main playing field, stood a giant torture contraption, made of steel and ropes and pulleys. And I was headed right for it.

In my quest to try new things and confront fear, I'd pushed

myself out of my comfort zone. As my running got better, I felt like I could do more, try more, avoid less. So I took more risks and went out instead of hiding at home. But I still sort of had a vague idea that I should do something that actually scared the crap out of me – not just things that made my palms a bit sweaty. So I did what any normal person would do and signed up to do a flying trapeze class.

It could have been a bungee jump, I suppose. Or a skydive. Or a fire walk. But they are all in limited supply in Central London and if I was going to 'feel the fear and do it anyway', I wanted to do it in a place that was easy to reach. Terror, yes. Long journeys, no.

So that's why I found myself staring up at a tower festooned with ropes and nets. To my eyes, it looked like a medieval torture device, and I began to feel fairly sick. The group session included some women who assured me that it was completely addictive 'after the first go', a man who'd previously given himself a black eye doing it – 'my own fault', he assured me – and a nine-year-old boy who looked raring to go. Nobody else seemed to have legs made of jelly. So I breathed deeply and pretended that I was as enthusiastic about throwing myself off a high tower as they all were. After some basic instructions, I was harnessed up and joined the queue to climb the ladder. The experienced people went first, jumping off the tiny ledge with no qualms, delightedly letting go of the bar and leaping to the next one like agile monkeys. As they connected with the second swing, they threw their legs over it and hung upside down, swaying back and forth. It looked so free. I was going to be sick.

The nine-year-old boy wobbled, and couldn't quite muster the courage. So I was next. I climbed. The ladder seemed to

go on forever. As I reached the top, a nice man clipped me
into the safety line, and coaxed me on to the wooden ledge.
At this point, I lost all my confidence. I didn't want to push
myself. It felt stupid and foolhardy, and I started breathing
too fast, aware that my vision was narrowing and everything
was getting darker – classic signs of panic. I stood on the
ledge for a few seconds as the instructor called up to encourage
me. Could I just climb down? Would I hate myself if I did?
The answer was yes to both questions. I tried another tack.
If I just flung myself at it, like I had with running, maybe
something OK would happen. Maybe it wouldn't end in
catastrophe as I always imagined. So I jumped. And it was
*horrible*. Stomach churning and too fast, and I didn't catch
the other bar and I had to drop to the net and laugh sheepishly. But I did it. Even though my body and my mind told
me not to. I knew enough that sometimes with anxiety, you
have to disobey what your entire being is screaming at you.

There wasn't much time to recover, as we were all lined up
again to give it another go. The nine-year-old braved it this
time, and everyone else nailed the leap. Except me. The feelings of dread didn't lessen, and I dropped to the net in seconds.
I think the instructors had realised early on that I was the
weakest member of the group, and extra rounds of applause
met me back on the ground. The entire group were incredibly
encouraging, and everyone had tips on how to connect with
the second swing. I had one more go, and I really didn't want
to do it again. But I didn't want to let down these nice people,
who were probably fairly embarrassed that I couldn't do what
a child had mastered. Up I went, wondering if I now had
vertigo, and reminded myself to google it once home. I jumped,
and I listened out for the instructor, who was yelling precise

orders at me. I grabbed the other swing, and locked my legs over. 'LET GO NOW,' yelled the teacher. But who the hell wants to drop upside down? So I swung for a bit, like Carrie Bradshaw does in *Sex and the City* when she tries the trapeze for an article she's writing (oh, you're too young, never mind), and waited. And then, suddenly, I did it. I flipped upside down and let the swing carry me by my legs. And it felt really fucking nice. So much so, I hung there until all the swinging had stopped, and dived on to the net below. I never went back, and I spent the next day in a fair amount of pain. But I'm no longer scared of the flying trapeze.

Like I've said about all my anxiety achievements, it wasn't a feat of bravery for the record books. It wasn't elegant, or something I relished doing. And I was really bad at it – even the nine-year-old looked at me with sympathy. But my self-esteem whooshed that day. I walked home on a cloud, enjoying every tree and bird and person I passed. It was an unrivalled feeling of accomplishment. And running had given me that. Running meant I could sail through the air for a few seconds. It's something I think about often, when I think about why I run. When I think about getting up early to do it, or worry that I'm not getting such a regular high from it. Because it's not just about the thirty minutes I manage on a wet Monday, or the fast pace I hit once in a blue moon. It seeps into every other part of my life, expanding them all, opening them up, giving me the self-esteem to go and do other things. I'm a running bore, that much should be obvious by now. But only because I found out that it could open up a whole life for me independently of it.

It sounds like a tenuous connection – going for a jog and then finding the courage to go on a trapeze. But I see that the line from one to the other is a straight one for me. Knowing that I could do a 10k meant I firmly believed I could swing upside down. I knew I could fly to New York for a job interview, and I could step outside my door alone without hyperventilating. I could have a day free of panic. Free of looking for the exit. Like Carrie Fisher said, 'Stay afraid, but do it anyway. What's important is the action. You don't have to wait to be confident. Just do it and eventually the confidence will follow.'[130]

Some people might laugh at the scale of the things I finally felt able to do – and I get that, when others might hop on a plane across the world alone without a second thought, or walk a tightrope for fun. But we all have our own levels of fear and our own yardsticks in the ground, and I have pushed past mine. I can't judge myself by other people's limits; I've spent too much of my life doing that and finding myself wanting. As Amy Poehler says about not judging choices made by others in her book *Yes Please*: 'Good for her, not for me.' [131]

Good for you if you can climb a mountain, or move to Malaysia alone for six months (like my brilliant sister did last year). I'll cheer you on. But I realise that pushing against my anxiety doesn't have to mean that we all have to have the same goals. I don't need to trek across continents to prove I'm not anxious anymore. I just need not to be anxious anymore. Like the lady said, good for you, not for me. It's a mantra to keep in your head when you start to judge other people, or try to compare yourself with them too much.

# 10K — PITFALLS AND DISAPPOINTMENTS

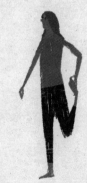

I'm running across the park, about 10k in, and it's boiling — it's a brutal summer which has given us no rain, and as a result, my back is a mishmash of sports-bra tan lines and my hair is getting lighter with every step I take. But I'm quite enjoying the dust and the throbbing sun — every minute feels like a challenge, and running in next to no clothes feels wonderfully freeing. I've been pushing myself on recent excursions, going faster, longer, taking fewer breaks. A period of unemployment will do that to you — running gives you purpose when you need it. I'm feeling pretty smug about it all, thinking about how I've made running a part of my life, how much it's now knitted into my make-up.

BANG! I've leapt over a dip in the ground, and my knee is screaming. I hop on one leg as though I'm trying to dodge molten lava, and clutch at my knee, as though a frantic rub will make the pain go away. But it doesn't, and I'm forced to hobble home.

I have 'runner's knee', which I must look at as some kind of horrible badge of honour, and not as a catastrophe which will derail all my progress. Exercises are prescribed, stretches, low-impact moves. I stare forlornly at my trainers when I set off to the swimming baths to do some lame doggy-paddle.

But I'll be back on the roads soon enough. My devotion to running goes deep, and perhaps I'll appreciate it even more when I'm allowed to head out again. Like a relationship that's gone a bit stale and needs a reset, I've decided to make more of an effort from now on. Who knows, maybe I'll even make myself try just one little race . . .

I like happy endings in films. I appreciate books where everything is explained and no character is unaccounted for. I would pay good money to bring Jane Austen back to life just so that I could know exactly what happened to the Bennet sisters later in life – even Mary. I don't like uncertainty. I don't like change. That's anxiety, and maybe also just who I am. But I know that life does not bring about these neat and happy endings very often. And I have learnt to appreciate the messy and complicated nature of us human beings. Stories don't have endings, they have peaks and troughs and long boring periods. And I would hate myself if I wrote a book which gave the impression that I was a mentally ill wreck with no future, until running made me some sort of superhuman who never faced another problem again. It's partly why I've never run a marathon, or taken on any other big running challenge. Because for me, there is no glorious end scene where I smash through the ticker tape and win a massive gold medal.

I hope I've been honest enough about the other things that have also helped me with anxiety and depression. I'm privileged – I have a family who have given me emotional and financial support. I've seen a good therapist who made me laugh and also taught me how to deal with my madder thoughts. I've taken prescription drugs – a fact I will never conceal from people again, as though there's a weakness in doing so. In fact, I'll fight you on it. That's how firmly I believe some people need them. I even fell in love again. Maybe for the first time properly. And with a man who's so kind and funny I can't believe he's not a monstrous trick sometimes. And he runs! Lizzie Bennet has nothing on me. I've been so lucky in lots of ways.

And yet running has been the hero in my story. The others have only got me so far – far enough to find the thing which helped the most. Or maybe it was running that helped me find the other happy things. Chicken and egg, I can't believe we're still using this phrase. But there have been times when I've assumed that running will be my magic beans, and erase all my worries, all my irrational thoughts, all my dark mutterings. And it hasn't, and that has taken some getting used to. When you think you find the miracle cure, it can be bewildering when you find out it has limits. Hugely ungrateful of me when you think about it, imagining that the simple act of running would inure me to all future sadness and worry. Especially when it's given me so much. Very spoilt.

So maybe it's worth being honest about the times when running has not helped me, or when I've taken it too far. It's vital to find the thing that alleviates your mental-health issues, and it's just as important to recognise that you will still have those issues. Don't imagine one thing can whisk all your symptoms away and pile them neatly in a drawer which you can lock up and walk away from. Running got me through many tricky periods. It ushered me through divorce, and job change, and moving house twice in six months, and it's a foil to my mental-health issues. But I still get nervous days, when my stomach churns. I still disassociate from time to time when

I'm worried about something. I sometimes have night terrors and wake up soaked in sweat, and my boyfriend rolls over, calms me down and changes the sheets. I fully expect that at some point in the future, I'll have days when I feel like I can't manage my anxiety, days where I spin out and want to climb out of my skin. But by knowing this, I can keep honing all the tools I have now to cope with these periods.

So, let me talk about my running failures, or maybe I should just call them pitfalls. I shall rank these from funniest to the least fun. Or if you prefer, shallowest to least shallow? And I can't bear to end on a negative, so I hope you'll indulge me some successes at the end too. Or just stop reading after the failures, that's cool also.

## I will never look nice when I run

Those bouncy, stylish people in neat kit with big fixed smiles? Not me. It's fine. Ish. Who cares anyway? Once you've gone past a minute, and your heart rate is up, you quickly forget to care what you look like. Sometimes I've glanced at myself in shop windows and seen a person who looks like she did aged eleven, red-faced, sweaty and with bad hair. People have backed away from me in shops mid-run, when I'm limping and gasping for water. But the more you do it, the more you realise that nobody is looking at you anyway. They're on their phones, and you have to swerve to avoid them. A person running at speed towards them is still not enough to get them to look up. You are less interesting than a GIF of a cat. Humbling huh?

## I will never not hate the first five minutes

It's important to remember this every single day I put on my trainers. I huff and puff as though I've never run before. I check the timer on my phone, and the seconds drag. My body will always want to give up and go home, and I just have to get through it and know that something magical will happen at some point about eight minutes in, where my body eases up, and my mind floats off, and it feels good. But it's important to keep repeating it, otherwise I'd never push through those first strides. If you feel like this too, just promise yourself you'll do one more minute and check again. By the time you do, the magic moment might have happened for you too. Full disclosure, sometimes it can take longer than five minutes. Sometimes it's more like fifteen. Sorry about that.

## I will never run longer than eighty minutes

I get too hungry and too bored. Sometimes running is boring. I feel like a traitor to my passion here, but it's true. Not every run is fun, or fast, or exhilarating. Sometimes it's a slog and you wonder why you bothered. I get jealous of those who can run miles without gnawing hunger or a wish to get back and eat a doughnut, but there it is. I'm not those people and I have to accept it. It doesn't mean I'm not a runner, I'm just not a long-distance runner. I think I still get the full joy, but if I push myself to go for five, ten, fifteen minutes more, I get shaky, slow down, and stumble. I've had to learn where my limit is. If you can run in total silence, I salute you. Otherwise, podcasts help, and music is brilliant if you find the right pace. (Puddle of Mudd sure kicked me off.)

## I will fall over a lot

Running has not made me elegant. It's just me, probably. I'm clumsier than most. My boyfriend eyes up any coffee cup I'm holding, waiting for me to spill it. I get angry that he assumes

I will, and then I do. And it's the same with running. I set off, knowing that today might be the day I take a huge tumble. And it often happens that I stack it, skid along the street and just suddenly hate running for a few minutes as I check out my bruised hips and grazed hands. Just in case you're like me, collective advice suggests you should try to tuck your arms in and roll to your side to lessen any impact. You do NOT want your wrists (or worse, teeth) to bear the brunt of your fall. Wear the resulting scars with pride, and tell people you got them in a duel or something.

### I can't let running take over my social life

I know how important this is, since it's happened before. I have an addictive personality (I'm not sure this is a scientific term, but for me it's an accurate description). I've allowed running to consume me at certain points, preferring to take a jog than to go for lunch, or dinner. I've left parties early so I could be fresh for a run the next day. It's a fucking stupid thing to do. Mental-health issues all thrive on loneliness, and choosing not to see loved ones so that you can run 10k on a rainy day is a mad move. But when I was first falling in love with running, and seeing it as the answer to all my problems, I became slightly in thrall to it. I still find it hard to say yes to engagements when I think it'll be tricky to fit in a run, but I also know I have to sometimes. I spent a holiday in Cornwall recently, and it rained every day. We were also situated on a fearsome hill, and I had to accept that running wasn't going to happen, and sit with it. It felt uncomfortable for a couple of days, but taking that break was more beneficial than any windy dark run would've been. I watched movies, and ate cheese and slept a lot. In other words, I had some balance. There must be room for all things. Running can't be the only bright spot in my life, nor in yours. And you don't have to go running on Christmas Day, unless you think it'll be a welcome break from your family (it might be).

## I will try not to use running to regulate my body shape

Again, this is something I've learnt from experience. In the early stages of getting into exercise, I noticed that I'd dropped a noticeable amount of weight. I started getting compliments on my cheekbones, on my stomach, and about how I looked so 'well'. Actually, I was a mess of heartbreak and self-loathing, but I couldn't deny that adding running to my life had meant a weight loss I hadn't anticipated. But it would have been surprising if I hadn't lost some weight, given I hadn't done any sort of exercise beforehand – ever. And the compliments felt nice, especially after a year where I'd received so few.

Instead of only thinking about what running could do for my mind, I also wondered how much more weight I could lose. I'd see how many calories I could burn by doing a run, and then make it longer, secretly congratulating myself on seeing jeans become too big for me, or noticing muscles I'd never had before emerge. This was a natural side effect of all the running; lots of people find that they lose weight when they first start out. And there's nothing wrong with wanting to stay in shape and keep trim. But maybe I had such a crappy sense of myself that I prioritised it too much, and lost out on some of the natural enjoyment I got from just meandering around, doing as much as my body dictated. I pushed it, going running twice a day if I felt I'd eaten too much, doing distances that made me tired rather than elated. It was too regimented, and a habit which was becoming addictive for a negative reason, rather than for the initial need for a break from the dark. It's not OK to be too tired to go out because you've run too far and not eaten the corresponding amount of food.

But I believed I was being healthy. After so many years of actively trying not to be active, I was moving, stretching, using my body. How could that be unhealthy? Except, of course, it was. Everything in moderation, so the saying goes. I always hated that phrase, thinking you should go all out with the things you love. But it's not totally wrong. Exercise twice a day if it brings you joy. Don't if you're forcing on your trainers and reluctantly shuffling towards the door because you ate a muffin. Or two.

Compulsive exercise is not a clinically recognised term, but there is enough anecdotal evidence to take it seriously. According to the US group, the National Eating Disorder Association, the warning signs include:

- Intense anxiety, depression and/or distress if unable to exercise.
- Discomfort with rest or inactivity.
- Exercise used to manage emotions.
- Exercise as a means of purging.
- Exercise as permission to eat.
- Exercise that is secretive or hidden. [132]

I ticked off a fair few of these behaviours. The worst being that I used exercise as a way to eat and not feel guilty – a thing I had never felt before, when I used to eat croissants as though there might soon be a world shortage.

I'd also get fidgety or annoyed if I couldn't run off my day, not just so that I could eat more croissants, but because I felt I only had the one outlet, and that a day without a run would be a day where I stored up anxiety. I think I was so scared that my anxiety would come roaring back on the one day I took a rest that I wouldn't let myself stop. But life makes you stop sometimes, and the fear and panic didn't immediately wash over me. That in itself was a revelation. I don't need to run furiously like a hamster on a wheel to reap the benefits (I once had a hamster which looked upon said wheel with disgust and went back to sleep, so I guess not *all* hamsters), and I'm not enslaved to running like I was to anxiety.

It's worth saying that this isn't a pitfall that everyone who takes up exercise will face. Most won't, but I tend to get obsessed with things, and I sometimes fall into a trap where I take things I enjoy to an extreme – the drawback here being that I can no longer enjoy them anymore. I spent a depressed period in my twenties eating family-sized bags of Doritos every day. I loved those chips. I can't eat them anymore, they taste like sadness. I ruined them for myself. Sure, this is a corn-based snack example, but it's a valid one nonetheless. Running is something I never ever want to have to stop because it's no longer fun, so I have to make sure I do it for the right reasons. Make sure you keep that in mind too. Ask yourself why you're really going for a run today, and make sure you have rest days, and time to recover.

## I will accept that running can't 'fix' my mental-health problems

I've touched on this before, but even now, I sometimes forget that I will still feel anxious and low, and I get surprised and resentful about it. I have been anxious writing this book, worrying about letting down a reader who might themselves be struggling with mental-health problems, and wanting to properly convey just how well I know the feelings. I worry about money, and jobs, and friendships, and sometimes I still veer off track and experience irrational thoughts which get stuck in my brain and frighten me. I have low days where I feel teary, or grey. Days when I wonder whether I'm going to end up back where I started all those years ago when I was almost housebound. But all these worries are a shadow of their former selves – an echo, or a faint imprint. They rear up, and freak me out, and mostly then they slink off again. Running is my shield, the activity I do to ward off these moments, but I can't inure myself to them entirely. Life will happen, and I can't always run it off. That's not a fault of running, or a reason to stop doing it. Instead, it's something I have to keep in mind, and when it happens, I try other things to boost the running. Sleep, eating well, seeing loved ones, trying breathing exercises. If you've read Hillary Clinton's book *What Happened* you'll know that, after the election, Clinton tried a stress technique called 'nostril breathing', or Nadi Shodhana Pranayama.

'You breathe through one [nostril], and you hold it, and you exhale through the other, and you keep going,' she explained. 'I can only say, based on my personal experience, that if you're sitting cross-legged on the yoga mat and you're doing it and you're really trying to inhale and hold it and then have a long exhale, it is very relaxing.' [133] [134]

I sort of raised my eyebrows at this, and then immediately tried it out for myself. And I found it relaxing! Other breathing exercises are perhaps more well established, and if they worked for Hillary Clinton after losing an election to DONALD

TRUMP, they might work for you too. Anyway, I try other things, and remind myself that, in the words of my mother, 'this too shall pass'. It's a message that seems hard to believe when you're in the throes of something dark, but it's helpful to repeat once in a while. Your mother probably had a similar saying, because mums always have well-worn mantras for sticky situations. Don't disregard them, sometimes they are all we have to hold on to.

Like me, Sara has experienced mental-health issues which have cropped up more than once. She's also had to accept that these crappy illnesses don't always go away fully – and she too uses running as a tool to fight off potential episodes, while also realising that it can only do so much.

'I was first diagnosed with postnatal depression in 2004, I was off work for six months. Since then I've had another four major periods of depression, two leading to more time off work. The last couple have been accompanied by quite severe anxiety as well.'

Sara told me that she used yoga and t'ai chi after her first bout of postnatal depression, and she knew that exercise helped with her symptoms, and she also recognised that stopping it usually signalled a low point: 'When I stop doing regular exercise it's a sure sign that things are starting to dip again, and then it's just a downward spiral.'

She took up running, and loved it almost immediately: 'Within about a week I got quite addicted and probably ran too much without really knowing how to support my body through that.' Sara injured her knee – please read the tips for getting started so that you don't end up with a similar injury. I know from experience how annoying it can be to get really into your running routine, overdo it, and end up out of action for weeks. She had another big episode of anxiety and depression shortly afterwards, and felt unable to venture outside the house without her husband, so the running fell by the wayside. But Sara missed it, and running found a way to lure her back. A friend, who understood her mental-health problems, scooped her up and took her out.

'She was an amazing support and just seemed to know how to deal with me. She used to come to my door, pick me up in her car, drive us to a remote hillside or wood somewhere, and we'd run for as long as I could, then she'd drop me back home again. It was a real lifesaver. It was winter too, so we ran in snow and ice and torrential rain, I tore my knee on barbed-wire fences and ran through ice-cold streams that chilled me to the bone. But it all made me feel alive again. And grounded. And that was something I didn't get in the same way from any other form of exercise. I'd also started to struggle with self-harm at the time, which provided another release from the numbness of depression and sense of disassociation I was experiencing. Running was a much healthier response to that, so it's probably saved me from a fair few physical scars too. In a way I guess that might be because running can be quite hard – it can hurt. So it worked well as a better mechanism for dealing with that side of things, the self-punishment.'

Because Sara knows that she'll probably face depression and anxiety episodes in the future, she has a healthy expectation of what running can do for her. 'When I'm going through a difficult time emotionally I have a bit of a love–hate relationship with running. I know it will do me good, but I don't have the motivation to get out there. And that in turn makes me feel worse because I then get annoyed at myself. I know that if I can just get my shoes on and get out there then after the first few steps I'll be feeling the benefits already. But it's making that commitment which can be hard, especially as my depression (on top of other, physical, long-term health problems) means I'm constantly exhausted! So I just have to keep reminding myself that even if I'm just out there for fifteen minutes, once round the block, and even if I walk half of it, I'll still feel better afterwards. Then each small run I manage to do builds up to have a more sustained effect.'

Every person who experiences low moments knows how hard it can be to motivate themselves to do the things which might help them. Sometimes the idea of even getting up to go for a run seems impossible. But Sara has the history to prove it'll help, so she gets up. She goes. And usually it works, but not always. 'Once I ran about a mile, then sat and cried my heart out uncontrollably at the side of the running track listening to Bob Marley's "Stir It Up" on repeat through my headphones! By the time I'd managed to pick myself up and run back home I felt physically and emotionally wrecked, but it also felt like I'd left behind a huge burden at that halfway point of my run. So it can be immediate, but those immediate effects can quickly wear off too, so I find I have to keep it up.'

I once found myself running through Hyde Park with tears blinding me, as I listened to 'Dancing on My Own' by Robyn, thoughts of how lonely I felt being spurred on by the lyrics. Like being in a bad montage in a movie, but with no surprise hunk to cheer me up at the end. Running can crack open emotions that you didn't know were lurking – those that in normal life you suppress or ignore. But they can rear up when you're out, moving, with an empty mind. I've felt utter ecstasy as I rounded a corner on the Euston Road, a strange moment where I sat laughing hysterically as I jogged in torrential rain in King's Cross, and a sense of immense calm creeping over me when running down an isolated French lane at sunset. These are not emotions I'm used to in my normal life, when I'm more likely to be feeling a bit irritable, or perhaps a bit sleepy. Such emotions can take you by surprise, like they did to Sara on the side of the running track, but I like to think that they were seeking a way to come out, to jolt you out of your routine and to make you feel more connected to yourself. As Sara says, when I asked her why she likes running: 'It quite simply reminds me I'm alive, I'm here, and I'm connected to this world.'

Sometimes anxiety and depression blunt our emotions, making us irritable, short-tempered, and filled with a sense of 'nothing'. Like me, Sara also suffers from dissociation, and running cracks open that sense of unreality for her. 'Sometimes with my depression I get so disassociated that I feel like I'm out of my body a lot – I even walk into door frames because I'm so dislocated from my body that I misjudge where I actually am in space. When I run I am fully present in the rhythmic pounding of my feet, the frantic beating of my heart, the wind against my face. So it really grounds me.'

Sara doesn't run every day, like me. She finds that she can pick it up whenever she feels a bad patch coming on. That's a skill I've not managed, but it works well for her. 'I've had bad patches since, and although I don't run through all of them, once I can get started again it does always give me that connection to "here and now" which is so important when my mood is just wanting me to be anywhere other than here and now! I'm in a pretty low patch right now, and realise I haven't been running for probably a week or two, which is a sign that I really should . . .'

Ideally, running should be something that you do when you feel like it – not something you feel like you must do, even when you don't really want to. But as Sara says, sometimes a low mood is a sign that you have to get out there again. As you get more comfortable with the notion that your mental health is something you need to monitor, you can start to intuitively know the signs which tell you that you might be about to enter an anxious or depressed period.

For me, those signs usually involve night sweats, disassociation, and a feeling that my body is being flooded with adrenaline. I get jittery, pacing about, and tapping my legs a lot. Those are all things I keep an eye out for, knowing that all together, they mean I'm stressed out about something. That might be a reaction to a real-life event, like moving house (I NEVER BELIEVED IT WAS AS STRESSFUL AS IT IS UNTIL I DID IT), but it also might mean my anxiety is acting up – and that doesn't always have an obvious trigger, sadly.

Sometimes, even with all the tactics and tools and understanding we can arm ourselves with to deal with mental-health problems, we can still be overwhelmed by an episode, with no forewarning and no rational or straightforward reason. A couple of years after I properly started tackling my anxiety and depression, I had to take a week off work because I felt like I couldn't get out of bed. I felt exhausted and spaced out, and I couldn't figure out what was wrong with me. I knew I was anxious and I felt bitterly disappointed that I hadn't stopped it from happening. I thought I was better now, and felt that there should at least be an obvious reason for my irrational thoughts and my churning stomach – and I spent many hours trying to figure out what it could be. But I never did set upon anything tangible. And eventually, I remembered that anxiety doesn't work with set rules. Human beings are always looking for an explanation, a reason, a meaningful excuse. But sometimes there just isn't one, and our brains really don't like it. It's uncomfortable to think that you can suddenly fall down a hole, and find yourself in a dark place again. But it's true, and when you accept it, it doesn't seem as scary as it initially might. It's not a failing, or a mark that you won't get better.

Progress with anxiety can often feel like a game of snakes and ladders, where you can quickly slide right back to where you started from. But that takes away all you've learnt about your illness, and relies on you forgetting about all the tools you've developed to deal with it. Even if you feel hopeless and despairing about yet another miserable or panicky moment, remember that you got out of it before, and that you can again. The internet is full of promises to end anxiety, and to cure it forever, but as the Anxiety and Depression Association of America warns:

'Beware of extravagant claims – instant cures, guaranteed results of never again having anxiety symptoms, revolutionary formulas, "natural" or unique methods or techniques that require payment . . . Just because it says "scientifically proven" doesn't mean it's true.'[135]

It can be tempting to search for instant cures (and believe me, I've tried. The amount of teas and apps and thought exercises I've tested out in the hopes that they will fix me is ridiculous). And they often include testimonials from grateful users who swear that their anxiety or depression has all gone, gone forever! That often means you feel useless when a calming tea does bugger all, or a yoga session doesn't stop your palms sweating and your heart racing. My advice is to step away from the internet when you feel real despair or sadness. There's some good stuff out there of course, but it's mixed in with rubbish, and in a weak moment you might be likely to listen to advice that won't help, or might make you feel worse. Also, reassurance is fleeting. Like popcorn, it never fills you up for long. It just reaffirms the need to seek it, if that makes sense?

So a good runner (and by good I just mean a person who enjoys running and wants to keep enjoying it) knows their limits and constantly checks in to make sure that it's still fun, and that they're still doing it for the right reasons. And if for any reason it stops working for you, don't be afraid to change your approach, or stop (GASP) entirely. Many runners get caught up in pace and timings. If this is you, try running for as long as your body enjoys it. Or just try something else. Sack it off for a bit and just walk aimlessly. Some of my most positive and calm days are those where I've taken the dog out for a long and meandering walk first thing. No psyching myself up to sweat, just a regulated pace, with more time to absorb my surroundings.

But sometimes, accepting the pitfalls of running frees you up a bit. Once I'd realised that it couldn't fix all my shit, I didn't suddenly want to stop doing it – I just realised that I'd have to do it in tandem with other stuff which also helps my brain. For me that means sleep, eating right, seeing family and work. God that sounds basic, huh? But sadly, and especially as you get older, that stuff is really important – especially if you're someone who 'enjoys' shaky mental health. Enjoys. I don't know why I wrote that.

Here ends my gloomy bit about how running will not make you glow from the inside or transform your personality from deeply cynical to bouncy and positive. Your pitfalls will be different (hey, maybe you're one of those maddening people who look fucking awesome when you run), but you'll find them. Just make a note of them and don't let them stop you. And please consider a phone protector if you're clumsy like me.

### Can we talk about my running successes now?

OK, good. In the interests of not being more self-absorbed than I've been already (all – through – this – book), I'll keep it brief. I list these successes here only to show what you can achieve if you decide to run too – if I could do it from an unfit beginning, then so can you. You'll probably achieve loads more. Also, do consider making a note of your wins – it's fun to look back at progress, and it'll gee you up on days when you feel like you've stalled or slacked off. I keep my runs saved on the RunKeeper app – I can add notes which help me remember why a certain jog was good or slow, and save routes I've enjoyed.

- I completed 5k in the midst of misery, with panic attacks threatening to strike at any time. That was the beginning, and still one of my proudest moments. It's also when I knew I'd carry on.
- I ran every day for a whole year. I'm not sure if I meant to do this, but somewhere during it, I looked over my running app and realised I hadn't missed a day and so, like Forrest Gump, I just kept going. It wasn't necessary, or always fun, but it was a tangible personal record that I can remind myself of when I get fed up with rainy, dark runs.
- I've run in every country and city I've visited since I started. Not only did I see the world in a different way, but it helped

me not to feel anxious or wary when leaving my comfort zone.

- I've encouraged others to run with me, when they were tentative or felt they couldn't. I hope that some of those runs begat other runners, or at least showed that they could if they chose to carry on.
- I've stepped up the miles, doing big, slow runs which loop the city and demand patience and a surrender to my feet. It's a different mental process to running a quick couple of kilometres, but I've tried to master it as best I could. Running 16k one afternoon recently made me realise that I can do it if I put my back into it. Sometimes running is entirely reliant on a stubborn refusal to stop. Long runs help you hone that skill.
- I'm still doing it. Nearly five years in, that's the running achievement I'm the most proud of. And I'll leave the bragging here, as promised.

# AND FINALLY . . . SOME TIPS FOR GETTING STARTED

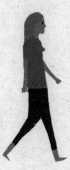

As I assume has been made crystal clear throughout this book, I am an amateur runner. A slow runner, maybe even just a bad runner. But I'm good at anxiety. I'm a master at that. And if you're the same, or just beginning to experience worries that seem to be mounting, you might want to give running a go too. If so, maybe my practical experience of starting out could help. Even if only so you bypass some of the pitfalls that I encountered. I should say that there are loads of books, blogs and apps for running too – there's the right advice for everyone, so if my tips don't seem right for you, seek out others, and don't just assume running isn't for you. It's far more likely that I'm just telling you what you already know – these are just my opinions, you can always find more. Which reminds me of that famous Groucho Marx quote – 'Those are my principles, and if you don't like them . . . well, I have others.'

- Exercise means having to overcome old habits of inactivity. We live pretty sedentary lives and it takes a lot to shrug off our normal routine. Running is hard work and can at times feel like the opposite of natural, even though it is. So make a schedule and try and stick to it. Otherwise your urge for five minutes more in bed, or one more Netflix episode, is likely to take over. These habits are hard to break.

- Don't buy masses of shiny new kit just yet. That urge will come later anyway, when you're in love with running, or at the least, when you know what you'll need. I didn't know I'd need a money belt until I started doing longer runs and getting stranded without cash for water or the bus. Running is a brilliant beginner exercise precisely because it doesn't need any special leggings or expensive equipment. I started out in an old tracksuit and comfy trainers. At some point, you'll need proper trainers – go and get fitted at a sports shop – I go to Runner's Need, but there are plenty of other places which will measure your feet and examine your gait. Don't worry about it yet.

- Go slowly. I mean it, as slow as is possible without walking. It'll feel ridiculous, and your body will instinctively want to speed up, but resist the urge. I started too fast, felt out of breath, got horrible stitches and quickly ended up with shin splints and a sore knee. Injuries this early in the game might put you off, and that would be pointless. Check your pace – download a running app which will tell you how fast you're on course to do a kilometre. Whatever that time, try and prolong it. When I cottoned on to this, I was losing steam after about ten minutes, and slowed right down – to the point where it took me over seven and a half minutes to do one kilometre. And that's fine, because you'll speed up as you get better. The important thing is to give yourself time to love it – and you won't do that if it hurts, or your body is screeching at you to stop.

- Download a beginner 5k app. This tip will not be for everyone out there — totally understandable if you want to run freely and not be dictated to by a strange and tinny American voice which will end up haunting your dreams. BUT — it can be brilliant for beginners who really have no confidence in their sporting abilities — and if you're already anxious or sad then let's face it, that's probably you — because the goals are really achievable and you feel like you're making tangible progress. I completed it in the allotted time, and the day I did 5k without stopping was utterly magical. I didn't feel overstretched, or furiously out of breath. I just felt invincible. And it doesn't hurt that by the time you finish the programme, you've run so much that most people get the bug and want to keep going . . .

- Take water. Most experts say you don't need to if you're doing short runs but for people with anxiety, it might help if you get panicky and need to stop. Take small sips, and wait until your breathing gets back to normal. Whenever I felt like I was panicking, or overheating, I'd stop and drink a bit. Then I'd realise that my heart rate was up because of exercise, not anxiety. I have a cool bottle which moulds to my hand and makes me feel like I've got a neon weapon. You can just get a normal one, whatever.

- Podcasts and music help. Again, not for everyone, but they help distract me when I get bored, or tired. More importantly, at the beginning, they made my brain concentrate on something other than worry when I ran. I still whack in my earbuds when I get anxious, or when a place is too noisy and I suspect my brain might start getting frazzled. I'm a big fan of Agatha Christie for that. Quaint murder, and the soothing tones of David Suchet. But death metal is also allowed.

- Take care of your feet. They are subcutaneous receptors – they respond to stimuli and transmit data about them to the brain. They are capable of doing so much more than you give them credit for. Respect them, give them rest days and if in doubt about your running form, go and see a specialist. Foot injuries will put you out of play, so please be careful. I have given up my beloved high heels for this very reason (and because uncomfortable shoes always seem to be designed by men who think it's fine to hobble, but that's a different book).

- If leaving your safe places makes you feel very vulnerable then start small, do a loop of your road. Run that road until you feel confident that you can go on to the next one. It all counts, and it's important that you don't push yourself too fast. Listen to your body. You can always venture out further when you feel more confident. I ran that little alleyway for ages before I pushed further, and I'm glad I did. I eventually got bored, and sometimes boredom is the enemy of anxiety. When you're no longer afraid, but just a bit fed up, you're less likely to be held prisoner by your irrational fears. I know of some people who have hired treadmills to start off in their own home, which is also fine if you have the space. I would've had to trade my bed for one, and I'm not sure that it would have been the comfortable thing to do in the long term. If it's too daunting to venture out alone, sign up a friend to go with you – or look for a local running club. Never be embarrassed to tell people that you're feeling a bit worried or that you need to stop – in her book about marathon training, Alexandra Heminsley said that in her experience, running makes people kind. I agree – so don't feel silly if you feel panicky, just explain it. Nobody will think it's weird or embarrassing.

- Remember that running does not have to mean marathons, endurance feats and six-packs. Some people will go down that route, and others will run around the park twice a week. As I've said, I'm in the latter camp, and I firmly promise that this option is fine too. However far you run is further than you've ever run before. What a brilliant thing. And it's brilliant if you decide to do a marathon too – but that's not the obligatory end goal. A 5k for someone with massive anxiety is a huge feat. If you compare yourself to other runners, you'll enjoy it less.

- Nobody is looking at you. I know you won't believe me initially, but it's true. You might worry about this if you suffer from social anxiety, and I completely understand the fear. Running feels incredibly exposing, overwhelming and scary to begin with. I ran in the dark, and stopped whenever I saw someone coming towards me. I didn't wear leggings for months, preferring to cover up with baggy sweats. I've thought long and hard about what I was most scared of back then, and aside from panicking in an unfamiliar place, my main one was being laughed at by strangers. I assumed people would mock me as I shuffled past them, point and make comments, realise that I was a total beginner, honk from vans. I've mentioned before that this is a common worry – especially for women, who also have to prepare for sexist comments while exercising. But nobody batted an eyelid. So much so, that I once fell over at the feet of a man on the canal path and he just carried on eating his sandwich. Cheers for that. I'm still angry.

• Running might seem like a mad thing to do when you've been scared and sad for so long, but to most people it's a mundane thing which they barely notice as they go about their business. You realise this pretty quickly – especially when you see that most people are glued to their phones and you have to swerve past them at the last minute. You might even end up wishing that people were paying more attention when you notice how annoying this is. The occasional goon will make a comment, but the great thing about running is, you're gone by the time you've heard it.

• Take time to see the beauty around you. I know this makes me sound like some kind of third-rate guru, but it's one of the joys of running. Your anxiety can make you introverted, never seeing what's around you, always forcing your brain to see negative, scary things instead. Running makes you look outside all of this, concentrate on your surroundings and use your eyes in a new way. Not just to spot people in your way, or know when traffic lights will change, but to see the entire space in front of you – be that a main road filled with people and traffic and shops, or a country lane with a few sheep. I've seen the beauty in all of it, purely from running. Nearly every time I go for a run, I stop to take a longer look at a building, or a poster, or a sunset. My phone is full of photos I've taken on my daily jaunts, of weird street names, of beautiful views, and of dogs I see along the way. The dog thing is weird, you don't have to do that. I look up a lot, at the tops of London buildings, which sometimes offer up strange architecture and beautiful ornate decoration. I run on the sunny side of the street and angle my face at the light, soaking up the warmth as I go. I promise that some of the things you will notice while running will stop you in your tracks, and you'll see things you'd never have seen if you hadn't run. I've grown connected to my home city in a way I never felt before I started running. I've pounded its pavements, and explored its secrets. And it's not just my own city – I try and run in every new place I visit. There's no better way to get familiar with an area, to feel its rhythm, to get to know its landscape.

- Running, just like everything else, is not going to bring instant relief. Just as antidepressant medication can take a fortnight to kick in, running might take longer before you notice any positive changes to your mind. Or not – I felt some darkness lifting pretty immediately. Teddy Roosevelt said that 'far and away the best prize that life has to offer is the chance to work hard at work worth doing.'[136] He was President of the United States, and I'm just talking about going for a jog, but then Donald Trump is President of the United States now, so the quote can still work here because apparently normal rules no longer apply in the world. It'll be hard. You might hate it for a little while, or even for a long while. But that doesn't mean it's not worth it. Sometimes when I'm running and it's cold and I'd rather be anywhere else, I rue the day I started. But I keep on. Because yes, it's hard, but I work hard doing it, and it brings me rewards I couldn't have hoped for five years ago. I've never committed to anything like I've committed to running, and that in itself is an achievement. If I was in the position to ask you – a stranger – a favour, I'd ask you to try it for three months and then reassess. Sometimes it takes that long to look back and see how much progress you've made. And you will have made progress, please trust me on that at least.

- Be kind to yourself. Cherish every little goal, make sure you recognise what it is that you're doing – you, a person who has a brain which has not always been your friend. Buy an ice cream after a run, have a glass of wine. Never berate yourself if you have a panic attack and need to go home abruptly. Running is not always a straight line (that would be boring). Sometimes there will be diversions and hold-ups. You can try again: it doesn't mean you've failed. You can't 'fail' running.

- Focus on what your body is telling you, but not too much. There will be times when you think you're going to start feeling anxious, and you must remind yourself that exercise brings out similar physical symptoms to panic – heavy breathing, sweating, a racing heart, shaky limbs. But this time, it's all for the good! You'll quickly get used to having these feelings in a positive situation. Feel your breathing settle into a rhythm, and notice how fast you get used to it. In a similar vein, take a note (mental or otherwise) of how you feel after each run – work out when is the best time of day for you to do it, and what you need to eat or drink before you head out. All of this will help you come up with some sort of running routine which can properly help relieve anxiety and stress.

- Have fun. I know it's obvious, but running shouldn't just be a joyless slog which you endure because you've heard exercise can be good for your mental health. Vybarr Cregan-Reid advised me that it was helpful to see running as 'not exercise', which I loved. 'Exercise is something that is mechanistic – you do it for a specific outcome . . . to get a healthy heart or to help with diabetes. Running is a lot more than a means to lose some weight. It's a multidimensional thing that's much, much bigger than just exercise.' Try to remember this. Try to run in whatever way works for you – whether that's for ten minutes, or doing hill sprints, or treadmill slogs or fun runs with mates. Sprint down a hill. Remember how you used to chase your mates when you were little? That childish abandon can be recaptured, no matter how long it's lain dormant.

I've said I can't end this book with just hope and joy and magic beans. But I also wrote a book about how running changed my life and released me from panic and misery. So I think *maybe* it's OK to document a few things that I've managed to do since that first short and sad run I took over four years ago. Life is tricky and gets diverted constantly, and we all stumble. I am the same. My life as a runner has not all been sunshine and motivational quotes (there have been no fucking motivational quotes at all – they are terrible things on the whole). There have been crappy times. There have been brilliant times. But the main difference between my life before I ran and my life since is that I have hope. And I have a life which is not always dictated by worry, panic, doom and depression. You can do so much more when those things don't sit on your chest and slowly squash you.

Some people might take my (small) achievements as proof that I simply grew out of my mental health worries, or that I was never affected by them too much in the first place. I assure you that neither is true. I was getting worse every year, and I felt almost totally despondent about the future. Anxiety rarely just 'leaves' you. Some people might be lucky and feel it float away one day, but for most of us it's a lifelong companion that we must learn to live with. But living with it doesn't mean enduring it, or giving in to it. It means finding ways to negate it, to dilute it, to push it back.

I have lived alone. Given that, before, I found my own brain too scary to sit with for long, this was a hard thing for me to imagine. I worried about being found dead with cats eating my face; I was scared that I'd be burgled, slip in the bath, set fire to the place (I used to carry candles outside when I went out, in case they magically 'relit' themselves). Mainly I worried about loneliness, and how I could be happy alone when I hated myself. But by losing the endless worry, I found myself underneath. It sounds ridiculous, but I used to not be able to articulate who I was, or even describe my character to myself. I just wasn't sure what was underneath the anxiety, which always stood out to me as my most prominent feature (that and my broken nose). Peeling that back (the anxiety, not my nose), meant I could see what else I was. And it wasn't so scary. I could be alone with my thoughts, and spend time without having others prop me up. I painted my flat. I decorated. I looked forward to nights in by myself. I didn't always need others to hold my hand when I got a bit anxious, I could adequately calm myself down for the first time. It was, for me, an extraordinary feat.

I travelled – on my own and with others. And I looked

forward to it. New experiences and big changes have always left me paralysed with fright – always looking for the potential catastrophe – but I've been able to go further and further away from the safety of home many times now, and it's joyful. Last year I managed New York for work, a place I was terrified of (skyscrapers and crowds and subways – oh my!), and I loved it. Being able to completely immerse yourself in a city you thought you'd never go to was the most exhilarating feeling. Walking around a strange place, with nobody knowing where you are, was something I could never have imagined I'd be strong enough to do. I look forward to new experiences now, without planning for the worst case scenarios around every turn. That approach, as you can imagine, can take the shine off a trip somewhat.

I changed jobs, and left the place that had been my safety net for eleven years. Safety nets are vital for people with anxiety, but nets can also hem you in. Trying something else was a scary but necessary step, and I had new faith that I could manage it.

I began a new relationship, one where I was open about my mental health, and enough of a complete person that I could enter into it properly, and without the need to control and limit where it went. It didn't hurt that this person I found was kind. Kindness enables you to face mental-health problems without being scared of the reaction. Without being told to toughen up, or get over it, or stop banging on. Tying two totally separate things like love and running together might seem like a fragile connection, but for me, it's one that's been made with a thread of reinforced steel. I could not have had another relationship without the strides I made – literally.

After such a massively disastrous marriage, my confidence

was shot. I sort of assumed that I could never have another relationship – should never attempt another. As though I wasn't meant for it – especially with all my obsessions, and worries and phobias. But slowly, slowly, I changed my mind, and maybe for the first time, felt like I was worthy of a relationship with another person. Enough to let go of the scars of last time, and fully jump in. What a complete and wonderful thing. I can't believe my luck – even now. A new relationship was sort of the last priority – I had to be sure that I could do everything alone before I tried to find a mate. I couldn't do what I did before, and rely on someone else to make me feel stronger, feel better. I had to be those things already. It's a measure of how over the whole 'starter marriage' I am that I sat across from my boyfriend at dinner last year and I proposed to *him* (he said yes, thank the lord).

So apologies for the slightly indulgent pat on the back there. These achievements are not much in the grand scheme of things. I've climbed no mountains, saved no children and won no awards. But I've done things that I never thought would be possible for me. I've widened my view of what *is* possible. And I've done it through running. Back then, that meant three minutes where I could break out of my brain, and escape utter misery. Now it means a morning run every day which can easily take an hour. It was hard in the beginning – both physically and mentally. I questioned why I was doing it every minute I ran. I felt stupid, unfit and useless. It's still hard. My feet would rather not be splashing in puddles, or hitting the unforgiving London pavements. I don't leap out of bed to do it. But I still do it. I venture out, and my head clears, and at some point I connect with my surroundings. My brain realises that there's more to the world than just my own fears. I see people, and beauty and mess. My feet connect with the ground and I am present in the moment. I flow, however awkwardly, however slowly. Thoughts pop into my brain, and leave just as suddenly. Nothing takes hold but the running. Worries can wait. More than anything, I've found a way to be alone without feeling alone. A way to be independent on my own terms.

Running takes faith. Faith that you'll be able to do it at all. Faith that your legs will know what to do, that you'll stay upright, that you'll get better at it eventually. It can be hard to hold onto this feeling, this hope – especially when it feels so hard in the beginning. But if you just keep going, you find the rewards eventually. You are a runner, and you weren't before. How fucking brilliant is that?

Mental illness takes faith too. Faith that you'll feel better. Faith that you won't sink into the abyss and stay there forever. And keeping that kind of hope going can feel impossible. And sometimes it hurts to be told you have to grasp it, when it seems nowhere to be seen. But as I've mentioned before, Emily Dickinson reminds us that hope is the thing with feathers. In fact, let's just read the whole thing. It's worth keeping in your mind on dark days:

> 'Hope' is the thing with feathers –
> That perches in the soul –
> And sings the tune without the words –
> And never stops – at all –
>
> And sweetest – in the Gale – is heard –
> And sore must be the storm
> That could abash the little Bird
> That kept so many warm –

I've heard it in the chillest land –
And on the strangest Sea –
Yet – never – in Extremity,
It asked a crumb – of me.

Faith, hope, whatever you call it. Cling on to it, however small it seems. Running was my hope. Or maybe running gave me hope, I don't know. But either way, it got me out of a lifelong cycle of anxiety and depression. It took me away from my shrinking safe space and pushed me towards a real life. It gave me faith in myself – if I could run, and run without fear, then I began to suspect that I could do more. A foundation to build on. A solid one – not built of sand, or in my case, panic. It is the one thing that has kept me on an even keel during some not very happy times. And it's all mine, I worked for it. I earned it.

It's not always easy. In fact, sometimes it's very hard. Because if I tell you to run for five minutes once a week, I don't think you'll notice big changes. It has to feel like work and it has to be done a lot and consistently. I don't much like the idea that 'everything worth doing is hard', but in this case it's true. We've come so far in accepting and understanding mental-health issues, but at times we stick too rigidly to the idea that there are a certain number of treatments which work, and so fail to explore other avenues. Running is another avenue for me, but it's no less difficult than any other method you choose.

Every run I do is different, even after all this time. Some are short, to shake off a burgeoning hangover (which only get worse as I get older, the warnings were true). Some are long, and whimsical, and I keep going just because I can. Sometimes I can go fast, and I feel tons of energy pulsing through my body. Occasionally, I get bursts of great joy and run down hills mentally screaming 'wheeeeee!' like a kid. Often, the runs I do are hard – but that's OK too, I know that they still matter. And every time I run, I get something from it. A break from the day, or time for myself, or I see something beautiful, work through a problem, slough off a niggling worry. I ran just before I wrote this, feeling spacey and tense after a fight with my mum. By the time I got home, the anger had gone. I might even call her later. My mind works through things as I run, even if I'm not aware of it.

Running is my relief. Relief after hard times. Relief during hard times. Your relief might come in a different form, but please do try and find it – don't stop until you do. Demand it, because you shouldn't spend another day in misery.

I promise that there are better days ahead. There are many ways to cope better with mental illness; there is support out there which you might not yet have discovered. I started my climb out of anxiety from a spot on the floor. It felt like an apt place for me – given that I'd never felt so low before. Gradually, I've made progress, shaken off the panic attacks, left behind the intrusive thoughts which I thought would send me mad with fear. I don't feel like I've said goodbye to mental-health problems – after all, the brain is like the body, sometimes things break, clog, slow down. But running is the thing I now know I can do to ward off the slew of symptoms that gripped me so tightly. It's as mundane as putting air in the tyres, or servicing a boiler every so often.

But more than that, it's made me happy. Not just from the flow, or the rush, or the instant energy boost it gives you. It's made me look out, instead of turning in all the time. And that made me see possibilities that I'd previously not known about. Things to be done; places to go; relationships to be built. And I've tried to grab them all. It's shaped my character and funnelled my anxiety into other channels. As Alain de Botton once wrote: 'The largest part of what we call "personality" is determined by how we've opted to defend ourselves against anxiety and sadness.'[137]

It worked for me. I have faith it will work for you. I'm going to shut my laptop and run now. Good jogging to you!*

---

* I told you I would.

# RESOURCES

Here are some resources that have helped me. If you feel like you need some support, they might help you too.

## Websites

https://www.mind.org.uk/ – Providing support for those with mental-health problems, and for their families. Lots of advice, facts and helpful links.

http://www.ocduk.org/ – A website dedicated to help adults and children with OCD. It has great blogs by people who suffer from OCD.

https://www.rcpsych.ac.uk/ – The Royal College of Psychiatry provides information, learning resources and advice on how to navigate issues like work and housing when you have a mental illness.

http://www.ptsduk.org/ – The UK charity which provides support and advice for anyone suffering from PTSD.

https://www.bacp.co.uk/search/Therapists – The British Association for Counselling and Psychotherapy can help you find a qualified therapist.

https://www.runnersworld.co.uk/ – A website stuffed full of amazing stories, tips and routes. Everything you need as a running obsessive.

https://www.nhs.uk/LiveWell/c25k/Pages/couch-to-5k.aspx – The hallowed Couch to 5K programme I've banged on about.

http://www.therunningcharity.org/ – The running charity I was inspired by: go and read about their amazing work.

https://www.thebodypositive.org/ – The site to go to for positive body discussion.

https://youngminds.org.uk/ – A charity specialising in mental-health matters for younger people.

http://www.activityalliance.org.uk/get-active/inclusive-gyms – A site which can point you towards gyms near you which can host those with disabilities.

## Apps

Strava – Maps routes and shows you where others go in your area, and lets you keep up with friends who also run.

Couch25K – Coaches you from the first minute of running all the way to 5 kilometres without stopping.

Runkeeper – Saves your running routes and times, and lets you record how you felt during every outing.

MapMyRun – Lets you record your run with a chip in your shoes if you hate taking a phone out when you exercise.

## Books

Adam, David, *The Man Who Couldn't Stop* (Picador, 2014).

Askwith, Richard, *Running Free: A Runner's Journey Back to Nature* (Yellow Jersey, 2015).

Austen, Jane, *Pride and Prejudice* (1813; Wordsworth Editions, 1992).

Bretécher, Rose, *Pure* (Penguin, 2015).

Burton, Robert, *The Anatomy of Melancholy* (NYRB Classics, 2001).

Challacombe, Fiona, *Break Free from OCD* (Vermilion, 2011).

Cregan-Reid, Vybarr, *Footnotes: How Running Makes Us Human* (Ebury, 2017).

*Emily Dickinson: The Complete Poems* (Faber & Faber, 1976).

Fisher, Carrie, *Wishful Drinking* (Simon and Schuster, 2008).

Gordon, Bryony, *Mad Girl* (Headline, 2016).

Harvie, Robin, *Why We Run: A Story of Obsession* (John Murray, 2011).

Heminsley, Alexandra, *Running Like a Girl* (Windmill, 2014).

Kessel, Anna, *Eat, Sweat, Play: How Sport Can Change Our Lives* (Pan Macmillan, 2016).

Mantel, Hilary, *Wolf Hall* (Fourth Estate, 2009).

Menzies-Pike, Catriona, *The Long Run: A Memoir of Loss and Life in Motion* (Penguin Random House 2016).

Morgan, Eleanor, *Anxiety for Beginners* (Pan Macmillan, 2016).

Murakami, Haruki, *What I Talk About When I Talk About Running* (Harvill Secker, 2008).

O'Sullivan, Ronnie, *Running* (Orion, 2013).

Otto, Michael, and Jasper A. J. Smits, *Exercise for Mood and Anxiety: Proven Strategies for Overcoming Depression and Enhancing Well-Being* (Oxford University Press, 2011).

Peterson, Andrea, *On Edge* (Crown Publishing Group, 2017).

Rhodes, James, *Instrumental* (Canongate, 2014).

Rice-Oxley, Mark, *Underneath the Lemon Tree: A Memoir of Depression and Recovery* (Little, Brown, 2012).

Rinpoche, Sakyong Mipham, *Running With The Mind Of Meditation* (Three Rivers Press, 2013).

Stossel, Scott, *My Age of Anxiety: Fear, Hope, Dread, and the Search for Peace of Mind* (Windmill, 2014).

Weekes, Dr Clare, *Self-Help for Your Nerves* (Harper Thorsons, 1995).

Young, Damon, *How to Think About Exercise* (Pan Macmillan, 2014).

## Something completely different

Sometimes we can feel so low or overwhelmed that exercise can seem like too much of a challenge. In these instances, be kind to yourself and don't push it. Instead, distract yourself from grim moments if you can. Here are some of the things I do:

**Audiobooks.** If you can't concentrate on a book without all the words getting blurry and your memory refusing to allow you to absorb even a sentence, consider audiobooks. Download something you've read before, to start with – I listen to a lot of Agatha Christie and P. G. Wodehouse because they're familiar and comforting. It doesn't matter if it washes over you, you'll dip in and out, and you may find it relaxing.

**Box sets**. In the age of streaming services, it's never been easier to take your mind off misery by watching eight episodes of the same show in a row. I'm not advising that you do this all day every day, but sometimes a good series can give you some respite from those anxious or sad thoughts. My go-to picks are *The West Wing* (punchy, dramatic and about a US president not called Donald Trump), early seasons of *Arrested Development*, and *30 Rock* for when I want familiar humour to soothe me.

**Cooking.** More specifically, in my case, baking. Making something with your hands can be incredibly helpful if you want to switch your mind off for a while. Try something complicated and fiddly for maximum absorption. There are tons of free recipe websites but my favourite is Nigella Lawson's site. Why not have a go at 'the Girdlebuster' pie? The name alone should intrigue . . . Find it here: https://www.nigella.com/recipes/girdlebuster-pie

**Gardening, sewing, painting, DIY.** These might make me sound like your nan, but they're all things you use your hands to do, and the doing *forces* your mind to concentrate on something other than your worries. Just try and make something. The result will hopefully make you proud, feel like you achieved something, or at the very least keep your brain occupied for a bit. I've painted some terrible pots, killed many plants and abandoned half-done clothes projects, but all of them really focused my mind while I was working on them. Gardening especially can feel like a chink of light – as my mother once said when I worried I'd kill anything I had to look after: 'Plants want to live.' Watching something determinedly put its head to the sky and bloom can be a reminder to keep living, even when it feels so hard.

**Go for a walk,** aimlessly, in a place where you feel happy – a towpath, a park, even your favourite neighbourhood. Focus on your feet and your pace – don't worry about speed or distance – just make like Forrest Gump and go until you're ready to head back. If you're feeling nauseous or full of anxious adrenaline, I promise you'll feel calmer after five minutes of strolling.

**Make a mental note of the things that work for you,** and if you feel a low moment looming, decide to bake that cake or dig out some paints. Collect your coping tools and let me know of any new ones I should adopt too. When you find what helps you, you'll be able to rely on these calming exercises forever, building on them, and knowing when to call on them. Good luck!

# REFERENCES

## 1K – Everything is Awful

1 https://news.harvard.edu/gazette/story/2008/06/text-of-j-k-rowling-speech/

2 J. D. Salinger, *The Catcher in the Rye* (1951; Penguin, 2010).

3 https://www.nytimes.com/1999/07/19/arts/to-invigorate-literary-mind-start-moving-literary-feet.html

4 https://www.ncbi.nlm.nih.gov/pubmed/19265317

5 https://press.rsna.org/timssnet/media/pressReleases/14_pr_target.cfm?ID=1921

6 https://qbi.uq.edu.au/blog/2017/11/can-you-grow-new-brain-cells

7 In Gerda Lerner, ed., *The Female Experience: An American Documentary* (OUP, 1992).

8 https://www.nice.org.uk/guidance/ph17/evidence/review-1-epidemiology-revised-july-2008-371243053

9 https://www.medscape.com/viewarticle/863363

10 http://www.ucl.ac.uk/news/news-articles/0813/22082013-Half-of-UK-7-year-olds-sedentary-Dezateux

11 https://www.gov.uk/government/news/number-of-children-getting-enough-physical-activity-drops-by-40

12 https://www.womeninsport.org/wp-content/uploads/2015/04/Changing-the-Game-for-Girls-Policy-Report.pdf

13 https://www.womeninsport.org/wp-content/uploads/2017/11/Girls-Active-statistics-1.pdf?x99836

14 https://www.nimh.nih.gov/health/topics/obsessive-compulsive-disorder-ocd/index.shtml

15 https://www.theguardian.com/education/2015/dec/14/majority-of-students-experience-mental-health-issues-says-nus-survey

16 https://www.theguardian.com/lifeandstyle/2016/aug/30/outdoor-fitness-parkrun-british-military-forces-project-awesome-parks

17 https://www.theguardian.com/lifeandstyle/the-running-blog/2018/apr/25/parkrun-makes-us-fitter-but-can-it-make-us-happier-as-well

18 http://www.manchester.ac.uk/discover/news/exercise-helps-young-people-with-psychosis-symptoms-study-shows/

19 https://www.psychologytoday.com/us/blog/the-truth-about-exercise-addiction/201504/how-many-people-are-addicted-exercise

## 2K – In Sickness and in Health

20 https://www.theguardian.com/commentisfree/2018/mar/07/mental-healthcare-patients-dying-reform

21 https://www.mind.org.uk/information-support/types-of-mental-health-problems/statistics-and-facts-about-mental-health/how-common-are-mental-health-problems/

22 http://blogs.bmj.com/bmjopen/2016/11/03/worried-well-may-be-boosting-their-risk-of-heart-disease/

23 https://people.com/archive/carrie-fishers-bipolar-crisis-i-was-trying-to-survive-vol-79-no-12/

24 https://www.mind.org.uk/information-support/types-of-mental-health-problems/anxiety-and-panic-attacks/anxiety-disorders/#.Wvxo45PwaRs

25 https://www.ocduk.org/how-common-ocd

26 Bryony Gordon, *Mad Girl* (Headline, 2016).

27 Eleanor Morgan, *Anxiety for Beginners* (Pan Macmillan, 2016).

28 http://www.nhsdirect.wales.nhs.uk/encyclopaedia/p/article/phobias/

29 https://www.nopanic.org.uk/agoraphobia-cause-and-treatment/

30 https://www.rcpsych.ac.uk/healthadvice/problemsanddisorders/shynessandsocialphobia.aspx

31 https://www.ptsd.va.gov/public/ptsd-overview/basics/history-of-ptsd-vets.asp

32 https://www.nhs.uk/conditions/post-traumatic-stress-disorder-ptsd/

33 https://www.mind.org.uk/information-support/types-of-mental-health-problems/statistics-and-facts-about-mental-health/how-common-are-mental-health-problems/#.Wv2Wa5PwaRs

34 https://www.ons.gov.uk/employmentandlabourmarket/peopleinwork/labourproductivity/articles/sicknessabsenceinthelabourmarket/2016

35 For more about *The English Malady* I recommend this BBC Radio 4 programme: http://www.bbc.co.uk/radio4/history/longview/longview_20031007_readings.shtml

36 https://www.theguardian.com/books/2001/aug/18/history.philosophy

37 https://www.nature.com/articles/143753d0

38 https://www.sciencefriday.com/articles/the-anxiety-riddle/

39 https://www.ncbi.nlm.nih.gov/pmc/articles/PMC5573555/

40 https://archive.org/stream/worksofthomassyd02sydeuoft/worksofthomassyd02sydeuoft_djvu.txt

41 http://www.appalachianhistory.net/2008/12/125-reasons-youll-get-sent-to-lunatic.html

42 Lisa Appignanesi, *Mad, Bad and Sad* (Little, Brown, 2007).

43 https://www.nhs.uk/conditions/generalised-anxiety-disorder/treatment/

44 https://www.nice.org.uk/guidance/cg155/update/CG155/documents/psychosis-and-schizophrenia-in-children-and-young-people-final-scope2

45 http://www.bbc.co.uk/news/uk-wales-19289669

46 https://www.pressreader.com/uk/daily-mail/20171229/281479276790129

47 https://www.theguardian.com/commentisfree/2011/jul/10/antidepressants-women

48 https://www.theguardian.com/science/2018/feb/21/the-drugs-do-work-antidepressants-are-effective-study-shows

### 3K – Suffer the Little Children

49 http://www.ucl.ac.uk/news/news-articles/0813/22082013-Half-of-UK-7-year-olds-sedentary-Dezateux

50 https://www.sciencedaily.com/releases/2017/01/170131075131.htm

51 https://www.rcpsych.ac.uk/healthadvice/parentsandyoung-people/youngpeople/worriesandanxieties.aspx

52 *The Diaries of Franz Kafka 1910–1913*, edited by Max Brod (Spargo Press, 2010).

53 Scott Stossel, *My Age of Anxiety* (Windmill, 2014).

54 https://www.sportengland.org/media/12419/spotlight-on-gender.pdf

55 Anna Kessel, *Eat, Sweat, Play* (Pan Macmillan, 2016).

56 https://www.womenshealthmag.com/fitness/a19935562/gymtimidation/

57 Alexandra Heminsley, *Running Like a Girl* (Windmill, 2014).

58 http://www.apadivisions.org/division-35/news-events/news/physical-activity.aspx

59 https://www.ocdhistory.net/earlypastoral/moore.html

60 http://www.bbc.co.uk/news/uk-england-merseyside-39702976

61 https://www.theguardian.com/society/2018/apr/26/mental-health-patients-seeking-treatment-face-postcode-lottery

62 https://www.theguardian.com/society/2016/feb/15/nhs-vows-to-transform-mental-health-services-with-extra-1bn-a-year

63 https://www.england.nhs.uk/mental-health/adults/iapt/

### 4K – Is It Too Late to Try?

64 https://www.nhs.uk/conditions/generalised-anxiety-disorder/

65 https://www.centreforsocialjustice.org.uk/library/mental-health-poverty-ethnicity-family-breakdown-interim-policy-briefing

66 https://www.centreforsocialjustice.org.uk/library/mental-health-poverty-ethnicity-family-breakdown-interim-policy-briefing

67 https://www.nhs.uk/conditions/generalised-anxiety-disorder/

68  https://www.theguardian.com/global-development/2016/
    apr/12/50-million-years-work-lost-anxiety-depression-
    world-health-organisation-who
69  https://www.refinery29.uk/best-quotes-for-your-20s
70  http://www.ucl.ac.uk/news/news-articles/0908/09080401
71  https://www.theguardian.com/commentisfree/2011/nov/06/
    charlie-brooker-becomes-a-runner

## 5K – Exercise is Intimidating

72  https://www.sportengland.org/news-and-features/news/2017/
    january/26/active-lives-offers-fresh-insight/
73  https://www.theguardian.com/cities/2017/feb/11/uks-cash-
    starved-parks-at-tipping-point-of-decline-mps-warn
74  https://www.rsph.org.uk/about-us/news/instagram-ranked-
    worst-for-young-people-s-mental-health.html
75  http://www.thisisinsider.com/fitspiration-social-media-
    negative-effects-body-image-2017-11
76  https://www.nhs.uk/conditions/obesity/
77  https://www2.le.ac.uk/departments/sociology/dice/documents/
    Sporting%20Equals%20Exec%20Summary.pdf
78  https://www.ncbi.nlm.nih.gov/pubmed/12213941
79  https://www.tandfonline.com/doi/abs/10.1080/00336297.201
    4.955118
80  http://www.sportingequals.org.uk/about-us/key-stats-and-facts.
    html
81  https://www.theguardian.com/lifeandstyle/2013/sep/16/
    exercise-fitness-disability-multiple-sclerosis
82  https://www.scope.org.uk/support/tips/practical/sport-fitness
83  http://www.activityalliance.org.uk/get-active/inclusive-gyms
84  http://healthandfitnesshistory.com/explore-history/history-
    of-running/
85  https://www.olympic.org/ancient-olympic-games/the-sports-
    events
86  Vybarr Cregan-Reid, *Footnotes: How Running Makes Us Human*
    (Ebury, 2017).

87 https://physicalculturestudy.com/2015/06/15/born-to-run-the-origins-of-americas-jogging-craze/

88 https://www.bmj.com/content/344/bmj.e2758

89 https://ajp.psychiatryonline.org/doi/10.1176/appi.ajp.2017.16111223

90 https://academic.oup.com/occmed/article/63/2/164/1376130

91 http://www.jneurosci.org/content/33/18/7770

92 https://uanews.arizona.edu/story/ua-research-brains-evolved-need-exercise

93 https://www.psychologytoday.com/us/blog/the-athletes-way/201211/the-neurochemicals-happiness

94 https://www.mind.org.uk/information-support/your-stories/i-think-i-might-be-dying-chapter-from-mad-girl-by-bryony-gordon/

### 6K – Pushing through Panic

95 https://www.nhs.uk/live-well/exercise/couch-to-5k-week-by-week/

96 Hilary Mantel, *Wolf Hall* (Fourth Estate, 2009), p. 182.

97 Thaddeus Kostrubala, *The Joy of Running* (Lippincott, 1976).

98 https://www.thecut.com/2016/04/why-does-running-help-clear-your-mind.html

99 Ronnie O'Sullivan, *Running: The Autobiography* (Orion, 2014).

100 Eleanor Morgan, *Anxiety for Beginners* (Pan Macmillan, 2016).

### 7K – Why Do We Run?

101 https://www.bhf.org.uk/news-from-the-bhf/news-archive/2017/april/new-report-assesses-impact-of-physical-inactivity-on-uk-heart-health-and-economy

102 Sakyong Mipham, *Running with the Mind of Meditation* (Three Rivers, 2013).

103 Stephen King, *Hearts in Atlantis* (Scribner, 2002).

104 Catriona Menzies-Pike, *The Long Run: A Memoir of Loss and Life in Motion* (Crown, 2017).

105 https://academic.oup.com/jcr/article/44/1/22/2970267
106 http://www.bbc.co.uk/news/uk-wales-40329308

### 8K – Know Your Limits

107 Haruki Murakami, *What I Talk About When I Talk About Running* (Harvill Secker, 2008).
108 Alexandra Heminsley, *Running Like a Girl* (Windmill, 2014).
109 https://www.theguardian.com/lifeandstyle/the-running-blog/2017/oct/21/ultrarunning-pain-cave-zach-miller-race
110 Haruki Murakami, *What I Talk About When I Talk About Running* (Harvill Secker, 2008).
111 Alexandra Heminsley, *Running Like a Girl* (Windmill, 2014).

### 9K – Listening to Your Body

112 https://www.gov.uk/government/publications/physical-inactivity-levels-in-adults-aged-40-to-60-in-england/physical-inactivity-levels-in-adults-aged-40-to-60-in-england-2015-to-2016
113 Damon Young, *How to Think About Exercise* (Pan Macmillan, 2014).
114 Haruki Murakami, *What I Talk About When I Talk About Running* (Vintage, 2007).
115 https://www.bluezones.com/wp-content/uploads/2015/01/Nat_Geo_LongevityF.pdf
116 Vybarr Cregan-Reid, *Footnotes: How Running Makes Us Human* (Ebury, 2016)
117 https://www.ons.gov.uk/peoplepopulationandcommunity/wellbeing/articles/lonelinesswhatcharacteristicsandcircumstancesareassociatedwithfeelinglonely/2018-04-10
118 https://www.psychologytoday.com/us/blog/the-art-closeness/201507/4-disorders-may-thrive-loneliness
119 Damon Young, *How to Think About Exercise* (Pan Macmillan, 2014).
120 https://news.stanford.edu/2015/06/30/hiking-mental-health-063015/

121  https://data.worldbank.org/indicator/SP.URB.TOTL.IN.ZS

122  Richard Askwith, *Running Free: a Runner's Journey* (Yellow Jersey, 2015).

123  http://time.com/5259602/japanese-forest-bathing/

124  https://medium.com/@ryancareyy/shinrin-yoku-how-the-art-of-forest-bathing-can-benefit-your-health-e7b37546d3af

125  https://www.ncbi.nlm.nih.gov/pubmed/19568835

126  https://www.mind.org.uk/media/273470/ecotherapy.pdf

127  Carl Jung, *Dream Analysis 1: Notes of the Seminar 1928–30* (Routledge, 1994).

128  https://www.huffingtonpost.com/hanne-suorza/how-i-run-with-mindfulness_b_7528280.html

129  https://www.cgu.edu/people/mihaly-csikszentmihalyi/

130  https://www.smh.com.au/entertainment/celebrity/stay-afraid-but-do-it-anyway-carrie-fishers-honesty-about-mental-illness-inspired-a-generation-20161228-gtiovy.html

131  Amy Poehler, *Yes Please* (HarperCollins, 2014).

### 10K – Pitfalls and Disappointments

132  https://www.nationaleatingdisorders.org/learn/general-information/compulsive-exercise

133  Hillary Clinton, *What Happened* (Simon & Schuster, 2017).

134  https://www.theatlantic.com/health/archive/2017/09/how-alternate-nostril-breathing-works/539955/

135  https://adaa.org/understanding-anxiety/myth-conceptions

### And finally . . . some tips for getting started

136  http://www.presidency.ucsb.edu/ws/?pid=24504

137  Penney Peirce, *Transparency: Seeing Through to Our Expanded Human Capacity* (Simon & Schuster, 2017).

# ACKNOWLEDGEMENTS

I didn't plan on writing a book about running. I didn't plan on writing a book at all. So I have to start by saying thank you to Joseph Zigmond, who read an article I'd written about mental health and thought that there might be a book in it. Once he'd ushered me through the initial stages, he handed me over to Tom Killingbeck, who has been totally brilliant throughout the whole process, never strict on deadlines, always encouraging, and instinctively right about tone. He helped make the process less daunting. Funny too, which helped when writing about fairly bleak things.

The rest of the team at HarperCollins have all helped me hugely – unravelling the mysterious stages of writing a book for me. Project Editor Lottie Fyfe, who put together proofs and worked on text design, Luke Brown, who copyedited the book and made my terrible grammar infinitely better, and Olivia Marsden and Helen Upton, who organised marketing and PR. I couldn't have picked a nicer group to help me write my first book.

I didn't have an agent when I started this book proposal. But over mulled wine at a Christmas party, I met Julia Kingsford, who generously offered to look through my contract for free and introduced me to her partner Charlie Campbell, who has been on hand to explain things, remind me of deadlines, demystify the language of the book world and, really importantly, send me advance money. They have both been incredibly kind and patient with me. And they have an office dog. Do visit them if you're looking for an agent.

To everyone who generously told me their stories for this book: I am still bowled over by your bravery, frankness and strength. Some of the experiences I was told in the course of writing this book reduced me to tears, and the fortitude and determination you all had to make things a bit better for yourselves (and for others) stunned me. You told me about your worst moments with mental illness in the hope that it might help others who struggle, and I hope that I have done you justice. Thank you all so much.

Thank you to my family, Lindsay, Alan and Lizzie, who have dealt with my worst moments with unending kindness and support – I wish everyone going through mental health issues could experience such an abundance of love. Nesrine, Archie, Maya, David, Miranda, who have all picked me up from time to time and never judged me. Barry, who helped fix me up and stop me being so scared, and lastly, Greg. You make me see new things with excitement and enthusiasm for the first time in my life. I love you pal.